OXFORD MEDICAL PUBLICATIONS

**Human Experimentation:
A Guided Step into the Unknown**

Human Experimentation: A Guided Step into the Unknown

WILLIAM A. SILVERMAN
Formerly Professor of Pediatrics, College of Physicians and Surgeons,
Columbia University
Christensen Visiting Fellow, St Catherine's College, University of Oxford

OXFORD   NEW YORK   TOKYO
OXFORD UNIVERSITY PRESS

Oxford University Press, Walton Street, Oxford OX2 6DP

Oxford New York Toronto
Delhi Bombay Calcutta Madras Karachi
Petaling Jaya Singapore Hong Kong Tokyo
Nairobi Dar es Salaam Cape Town
Melbourne Auckland

and associated companies in
Beirut Berlin Ibadan Nicosia

Oxford is a trade mark of Oxford University Press

Published in the United States
by Oxford University Press, New York

First published 1985
Reprinted 1986
First issued in paperback 1986

British Library Cataloguing in Publication Data
Silverman, William A.
Human experimentation: a guided step into
the unknown.——(Oxford medical publications)
1. Medicine, Clinical——Research   2. Human
experimentation in medicine
I. Title
615'.7   R853.H8
ISBN 0-19-261499-1
ISBN 0-19-261636-6 (pbk)

Library of Congress Cataloging in Publication Data
Siverman, William A.
Human experimentation.
(Oxford medical publications)
Bibliography: p.
Includes index.
1. Human experimentation in medicine. 2. Medicine,
Clinical——Research. I. Title. II. Series. [DNLM:
1. Ethics, Medical.   2. Human experimentation.
W 20.5 S5872h]
R853.H8S57   1985   174'28   84-27162
ISBN 0-19-261499-1
ISBN 0-19-261636-6 (pbk)

Printed and bound in
Great Britain by Biddles Ltd
Guildford and King's Lynne

I dedicate this book to my teacher
RICHARD L. DAY
He observed that a student is
someone who thinks otherwise. And
he taught that it is dangerous to
treat this healthy state of mind.

Preface

There is no question that medicine has made unprecedented strides in recent years, but an increasing number of voices now ask, Where is medicine going? The goal was stated succinctly in 1952 by Nobel laureate MacFarlane Burnet:

The aim of medicine in the broadest sense is to provide for every human being, from conception to death, the greatest fullness of health and length of life that is allowed by his genetic constitution and by the accidents of life.

In reviewing the historic development of medical research as a means to further this end, he found evidence that scientific investigation in this field had, indeed, grown out of human need. But he expressed concern that the activity (i.e. the systematization of methods for the most effective satisfaction of human desires) might lose contact with social aims.

In the years since Burnet's thoughtful analysis, a powerful new methodological tool in medical research has been perfected—the randomized clinical trial. This development grew out of an earlier refinement, random order of assignments, in biological experiments on conditions undergoing concurrent comparison. The new strategy, first in preclinical and later in bedside experimentation, led to a leap forward that has been compared, by Mervyn Susser of Columbia University, to the abrupt advance following the invention of the microscope. But unlike other tools in medical research, the use of the randomized clinical trial requires the full co-operation of relatively large numbers of human beings. The nature of this investigative 'instrument' links it inextricably with social considerations.

In the period immediately after World War II, many new treatments were introduced to improve the outlook for prematurely-born babies. (These infants accounted for the largest number of deaths in the days and weeks after birth.) Over the next few years it became painfully clear that a number of changes in caretaking practices had produced completely unexpected harmful effects. The most notable of these tragic clinical experi' nces was an 'epidemic' of blindness, retrolental fibroplasia, in the years 1942–54. The disorder was found to be associated with the way in which supplemental oxygen had come to be used in the management of incompletely developed newborn babies. The twelve-year struggle to halt the outbreak provided a sobering demonstration of the need for planned evaluation of all medical innovations before they are accepted for general use. One observer noted that when the value of a treatment, new or old, is doubtful, there may be a higher moral obligation to test it critically than to continue to prescribe it year-in, year-out, with the support merely of custom or wishful thinking. Formal strategies for clinical testing evolved to fulfill this newly-prominent obligation.

During this period of 'awakening' (in the early 1950s) I began to use the (then) recently developed format of the randomized clinical trial as a tool for evaluating some of the many new treatments for premature infants in The Babies Hospital at Columbia University. I was soon convinced of the utility of the schematic approach, despite the practical difficulties. Repeated experience provided impressive demonstrations of the intrinsic caution and fairness of this approach: scientific *and* democratic principles proved to be complementary (not antithetical!). I fully expected that the new techniques would be accepted rapidly, but my prediction was quite wrong. As the years have rolled by, opposition to pre-planned human experimentation has increased. The objections are in complete disaccord: some have argued that the rigorous demands of randomized trials delay the introduction of urgently needed treatments to relieve suffering; others have accused investigators of proceeding too rapidly (i.e. by exposing patients to unproven 'experimental' treatments). The incongruity of these positions and the rising clangor of the debates have convinced me that there is an alarming and ever-widening communication gap which separates medical inquirers from the rest of society. The message that must be widely broadcast is this: observation and experiment are fundamentally different kinds of operations.

The way in which doctors attempt to apply the experimental format in the design of human studies is set out in the pages which follow. In this volume, I have leaned heavily on my own experiences with treatment trials involving newborn babies. I must explain that the examples in this field of medicine are by no means unique. I believe, however, that studies involving helpless neonates call attention to some of the most difficult stumbling blocks which stand in the way of widespread acceptance of the need for planned studies. Additionally, there is a need to be more critical about the quality of evidence in matters relating to infants and children than in any other province in medicine. If evidence misleads in the case of interventions for adult patients—particularly those beyond the age of reproduction—the long-term global consequences of error are relatively trivial. Since ours is the only species on the planet which has achieved rates of newborn survival which exceed 90 percent, it seems to me we must demand the highest order of evidence possible before undertaking widespread actions that may affect the full life times of individuals in the present as well as in future generations. Here a strong case can be made for a *slow* and *measured* pace of medical innovations. (Premature dissemination of a new medical technique, before evaluation by carefully designed clinical trials, has been likened by Eugene Braunwald of Harvard University to a genie who has escaped from a bottle—it is virtually impossible to undo the confusion resulting from such unrestrained therapeutic exuberance.) Finally, I have focused on a relatively few examples of medical problems (repeated reference is made to the retrolental fibroplasia experience) in the hope of lightening the semantic burden for the non-medical reader who must cope with unfamiliar medical terms and concepts in addition to those concerned with research methodology—the central issue in this book.

The philosophic outlook called 'critical rationalism' is the epistemological underpinning of the scientific attitude. A fundamental insight of this view of the world is that we can learn from our mistakes. Critical examination of knowledge claims is the only way we have of detecting our blunders and harnessing them for useful purposes. I have emphasized this outlook which is the root premise for the kind of experimentation seeking to discriminate between possibilities. In addition I have stressed the design of clinical experiments and the logical foundation of statistical methods rather than the arithmetic operations used in the analyses of outcomes in clinical trials. Workable clinical experiments simply cannot be designed with lofty detachment from the frustrating details of the real world. In the pages of this book, I have made an effort to dispel the simplistic notion that the use of scientific rules of evidence in human experimentation implies that there is a fixed set of directions that may be applied mechanically to test a given question. The disturbing assumption of such a myth is that if you go through the motions attributable to science, then science will result. (Such operations, sociologist Erving Goffman once pointed out, are reminiscent of the experiments children perform with toy sets: 'Follow the instructions and you can be a real chemist, just like the picture on the box.')

The phrases 'dramatic breakthrough', 'miracle drug', 'life-saving discovery', and the like are often applied to the results of medical research; there is, consequently, an understandable belief that only money and national resolve stand in the way of any rapid solution to major medical problems. It may come as a rude shock to read my account of a catalogue of obstacles that must be overcome to make very modest gains in improving the outlook for most of our afflictions. It would be well, I suggest, for those who are impatient with the fact that a medical millennium is

Contents

1 'Knowing' in medicine

For countless ages, the ailing have turned to 'healers' who profess to know how to bring about relief and cures. The affected give little thought to the gnawing question, *How* do they know? Indeed, most of us, when ill, prefer to avoid raising such doubts for conscious consideration. Even a shaman who engages in deliberate deceptions has been known to turn to other shamans for treatment when he himself is sick. However, once the element of blind faith is set aside, the question of 'knowing' in medicine is not different from the general question, How do we know what we know about the natural world?

Knowledge grows by the solution of problems; the primitive approach to solutions is the trial-and-error method used by all living forms in the course of adaptation. Since the number of errors in random explorations is large, the crude method is slow and costly. The probings of humankind and of some animals gain in efficiency as they are guided by abstract reasoning. However, the major human advantage is that of time-binding; each generation can begin where the previous one left off. Unfortunately, the enormous power of this faculty is blunted when the received messages discourage fresh explorations. For example, at the time of a solar eclipse, some South Pacific natives blow whistles, shout, and beat drums to frighten the moon into disgorging the sun. When the intervention is challenged, the leaders reply, in effect, why change, it works.

A HERITAGE OF AUTHORITARIANISM

Uncritical reliance on past experience, *post hoc ergo propter hoc* reasoning, and veneration of dogma proclaimed by authoritative figures, were all embodied in a form of medical thought known as Galenism. Galen (AD 138–201) codified a system of medicine that endured without challenge in the Western world for about sixteen centuries. It was based on his vast experience as a physician in Rome, and on dissections and experiments in animals.

The general approach was teleologic: Nature acts with perfect wisdom, he held, and does nothing uselessly. Galen wrote extensively and made statements with impressive self-confidence about virtually every medical topic. His words were regarded as immutable by worshipful followers.

When Andreas Vesalius, a 16th century Belgian physician, first dissected a human heart and did not find 'pores', said by Galen to perforate the septum separating the ventricular chambers, the Belgian assumed the openings were invisible to the eye. Some years later, with his faith in authority shaken, he declared dramatically that 'pores' did not exist. Vesalius' book describing dissections of the human body appeared in 1543. It undermined the foundations of Galen's pronouncements by showing that the long-accepted descriptions of human anatomy were incorrectly set down. The Galenists, who formed the majority of university physicians, vehemently denied the truth of the new statements.

Galen's erroneous views that blood flowed to and fro in a tide-like movement within arteries and veins were not upset until the 17th century. The announcement of the discovery of the circulation of the blood by an English physician, William Harvey, in 1628, met with violent opposition. Even when it was admitted, grudgingly, that Harvey might be right, a defender of the established view wrote that if the new findings did not agree with Galen, the discrepancy should be attributed to the fact that Nature had changed; one should not admit that the master had been wrong.

An aphorism ascribed to Galen reveals the kind of invulnerability claimed by physicians for hundreds of years:

All who drink of this remedy recover in a short time, except those whom it does not help, who all die. Therefore, it is obvious that it fails only in incurable cases.

GROWTH OF SCEPTICISM

Western medicine's progress from mystical certainty to scientific uncertainty began with the challenges to Galenism. And the spirit of doubt spurred an exponential growth in inquiry that has continued to the present day. In the short time since World War II, an enormous amount of descriptive information has been collected concerning the constituent parts of the human body down to the smallest subcellular and molecular units. Vital functions and specific disorders are now described in the mechanistic terms of biochemistry and physiology, and a powerful array of drugs and physical agents have been developed to modify physiological and pathological processes.

Much of this has come about as the result of ingenious technical developments which have permitted never-before-possible observations and measurements. But, more significantly, never-before-challenged hypotheses have been questioned and formal rules of scientific evidence have been applied with increasing frequency in tests of hypotheses.

I underline the importance of this shift in emphasis (from collecting observations to testing ideas) because there is a common belief that the scientific method is an engine-like operation for the assembly, classification, and interpretation of facts about the material world. In the pages that follow, I will dwell repeatedly on the limitations of the observations-only approach in medicine. Here I wish to point out the curious origin of the incomplete view of how we set out to make sense out of information. The roots extend back to the time of William Harvey in the ideas of one of his influential patients, Francis Bacon, a Lord High Chancellor in 17th century England.

The millenarian view

The notion that wholesale collections of observations about natural events can provide perfect knowledge about the world can be traced to an interpretation of biblical text. The inspiration came from the Book of Daniel, Chapter 12, in which the prophet described the final state of the world before the millennium. In Verse 4 it is foretold that at the time of the end '... many shall run to and fro, and knowledge shall be increased'.

These lines of scripture, British historian Charles Webster has shown, played a surprising role in the development of science and medicine, for they were used by Bacon and his Protestant co-religionists to resolve a basic dilemma facing them in the early 1600s.

If Man originally fell owing to his pursuit of knowledge, how was it *now* possible for him to seek worldly enlightenment without falling from grace? Bacon argued that all knowledge must recognize and be guided by the primacy of religion. Probing what he defined as 'secondary causes' for utilitarian purposes would, therefore, incur no risk of transgression. Instead, these mundane explorations would glorify God and restore Man's dominion over Nature.

The notion of restoration was central to Bacon's thesis; the idea was to recapture intellectual attributes lost by Adam at the time of the Fall. The pursuit would hasten the coming of the millennium, a return to conditions of life associated with the Garden of Eden. According to the prophet Daniel, Man was destined to regain a position of dominance. Each step to increase knowledge was a move toward the millennial condition. Bacon proposed '... to extend the power and dominion of the human race over the universe'.

Bacon's inductive method

The project was set out in Bacon's book entitled *Instauratio Magna* which appeared in 1620. The great restoration of Man through science was to be accomplished through a new method of research called *Novum Organum* (also hailed as 'True Directions Concerning the Interpretation of Nature').

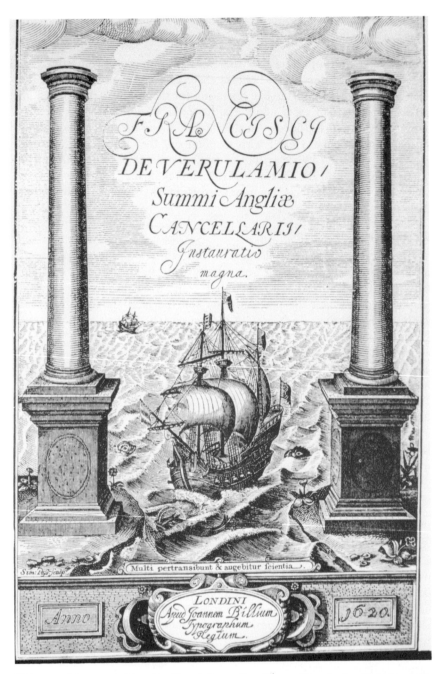

Title page of *Instauratio Magna* by Francis Bacon (first Baron of Verulam) published in 1620. The pregnant line from Daniel 12:4 appears here in Latin—*multi pertransibunt et augebitur scientia* ('many shall run to and fro and knowledge shall be increased'). Note the symbolism of the two Pillars of Hercules at the entrance to the Mediterranean Sea; these marked the farthermost limits of the habitable world in the minds of the ancients. Here Bacon indicates voyages of exploration beyond the time-honored limits.

The improved plan of discovery consisted of deriving laws from collections of observations—the method of induction. Bacon was convinced that a very diligent dissection of the world would provide the means for *completely* understanding it.

He also advised that observers invent experiences without waiting for Nature to act. And he argued that his scheme would have the effect of transferring the business of finding the pattern-of-particulars from the mysterious operations of the imagination to a logical procedure. It should be possible, therefore, to develop a mechanical course of action to discover laws governing any aspect of natural phenomena. He said, 'My way of discovering sciences leaves little to individual excellence, because it performs everything by the surest rules and demonstration.'

Bacon was certain the co-operative effort of large teams of researchers would lead to the speedy discovery of *everything there is to know*.

The spirit of Galilean experimentation

Galileo expert Stillman Drake has recounted the story of an argument concerning floating objects in water that began in the summer of 1611 at a small meeting in Florence. There was a discussion about condensation of matter by cold—ice was mentioned as an example. Galileo said ice is rarified water and merely appears to be dense. Since it floats, he argued, ice must be lighter than water. A professor of philosophy explained the floating of ice by its broad and flat shape; it is unable to cleave the surface resistance of water and this keeps it afloat. The argument went on for months; finally, the opponents met to sign an agreement fixing the conditions of a contest which could be judged by referees.

The defender of the shape-theory planned to use pieces of ebony, some in the form of thin chips and some in spherical and cylindrical shapes. Since the flat pieces could be floated while the balls and cylinders would invariably sink, this was to be offered as experimental proof that shape was the only factor which determined the floating or sinking of bodies in water. Galileo, on the other hand, proposed that different shaped pieces of ice and of ebony should be submerged in water and then released.

The contest never took place because the shape defender never appeared at the appointed time. But the spirit of Galileo's approach is perfectly obvious. He proposed a critical experiment that placed the rarified water explanation at maximum risk—it was designed to allow observers to make a clear choice between competing theories concerning the floating of objects in water.

Galilean experimentation

Bacon's inductive approach was fundamentally different from the method of research clarified by his contemporary, Galileo Galilei. The Florentine astronomer and physicist recognized that there are usually competing explanations for a phenomenon and he tried to devise tests which could discriminate between possibilities. Bacon advised that experiments (invented experiences) be carried out merely to increase the supply of observations for the engine of induction; Galileo's experimental design appealed to experience for the express purpose of testing some postulated law.

Most important, the critical methodology was open-ended; it discarded the millennial idea of completeness of observations and experience because no earthly criterion of 'completeness' could be envisioned. The deductions from a mathematical formula or an hypothesis were subjected to an ordeal (*il cimento*); if they failed the test, the experimenter devised fresh experiments in the light of what had already been observed.

This method of discovery depended (as it does today) on an essential element—the creative imagination of the experimenter. It was accepted that the concept of 'knowing' has a provisional quality; there is uncertainty about the durability of explanations. And it followed that there must be tentative acceptance of only those theories which have survived rigorous critical tests.

'The observer listens to nature; the experimenter questions and forces her to unveil herself.'

Georges Cuvier

Endurance of inductivism

The founders of the Royal Society of London made it clear that they acquired the concept of a systematic investigation of the natural world from Bacon. But the Fellows of the Society changed over to the approach of Galileo, almost without comment on the difference between the two versions of the scientific method.

The curious thing about all of this is that inductive logic became established as a tradition in science. Despite the shortcomings recognized at the very start and criticism of this type of reasoning by philosophers from David Hume to Karl Popper, the idea persisted that knowledge grows by collecting facts on a grand scale. What is even more amazing about the durability of inductivism is the clear evidence that it was not used by those who made the most important advances in science and medicine. (Harvey was not influenced by his patient; he said of Bacon, 'He writes Philosophy like a Lord Chancellor.')

Biologist Peter Medawar examined the paradox in which researchers pay lip reverence to a style of investigation which they do not use and cannot authenticate from their own experience. 'Sciences which remain at Bacon's level of development,' he pointed out, '... amount to little more than academic play.'

EXPERIMENTAL METHODS IN CLINICAL STUDY

Over 100 years ago the French physician and physiologist, Claude Bernard, recognized that developments in the basic sciences were gradually turning medicine 'toward its permanent scientific path'. Nonetheless, there was an unresolved problem; physicians were slow to adopt the method of investigation common to the sciences. He noted, for example, that they appeared unwilling to concede the important distinction between the analytic power of observation and that of experiment.

Bernard explained the principles that form the basis of experimental reasoning in his classic treatise, *An Introduction to the Study of Experimental Medicine* published in 1865. He stressed that 'Gaining experience and relying on observation is different from making experiments and [recording] observations.' And he made strong arguments for 'precise reasoning based on an idea born of observation and controlled by experiment'. Bernard called for a shift to critical (Galilean) methods in medical research.

His words had, and continue to have, a very wide influence on medical thought. Nonetheless, it would be misleading to ignore the fact that the resistance he sought to overcome has not yet disappeared. Medicine still struggles with a double standard of credulity in its search for understanding and effective action.

Faltering support for scientific rigor

Preclinical studies in laboratories are carried out under the watchful eyes of referees—tough critics who insist that rules of evidence be strictly observed. A constantly remodelled body of biomedical evidence has been assembled, and it serves as the fertile source of rational proposals for everyday applications in medical practice.

The next step, an experimental test of predicted effects of interventions in groups of patients, falters because of a block well known to Bernard. 'Many physicians attack experimentation,' he said, 'believing that medicine should be a science of observation, but physicians make therapeutic ex-

---

An eighteenth century controlled trial

'On the 20th of May, 1747, I took twelve patients in the scurvey aboard the Salisbury at sea. Their cases as similar as I could have them ... Two of these were ordered a quart of cider a day. Two others took twenty five gutts of elixir vitriol ... Two others took two spoonfuls of vinegar ... Two were put under a course of sea water. Two others had each two oranges and one lemon given them each day ... The two remaining took the bigness of a nutmeg ... The consequence was the most sudden and visible good were perceived from the use of the oranges and lemons.'

James Lind, 1753

periments daily on their patients so this inconsistency cannot stand careful thought. Medicine by its nature is an experimental science,' he continued, 'but must apply the experimental method systematically.'

The practical difficulties of carrying out this hundred-year-old advice are considerable. Unfortunately, there is no other way to obtain evidence of an order which approaches the rigorously objective kind we seek by scientific inquiry in all other areas of the material world. The rules of scientific evidence cannot be repealed by pleading hardship.

Impatience with delays

There are understandable, if not strictly logical, reasons for the reluctance to submit hopeful treatments to experimental tests in matters involving the well-being and the lives of our fellow humans. The slow, painstaking steps and the scepticism which underly the reasoning seem niggling in the face of suffering and rapidly progressing illness. After basic studies concerning isolated phenomena have been rigorously battle-tested, there is an understandable temptation to translate the hard-won information into practical action as quickly as possible. The powerful urge is given a boost by the machinery of present day mass communication which needs to be fueled by an endless flow of miracles.

It is probably unnecessary to seek further for an explanation of the ambivalence which characterizes attitudes toward the experimental approach in modern clinical research. For it is hard to deny that doubt is unwelcome at the bedside; we have a deep-seated yearning for magical cures.

Stepping into the unknown

Despite dramatic modern victories, failed innovations continue to outnumber successes in medicine. Moreover, the consequences of therapeutic error were relatively insignificant until the modern era. For example, when Galen advocated 'Mucilage of Holihock' for the cure of piles, few patients were injured.

Like weapons in the modern arsenals of war, therapies have become exceedingly powerful and the potential for harm on a very wide scale has escalated accordingly. Spectacular therapeutic disasters have made it clear that informal let's-try-it-and-see methods of testing new proposals are more risky now than ever before in history. Since there are no certainties in medicine, it must be understood that every clinical test of a new treatment is, by definition, a step into the unknown.

The community at large (and specifically lawyers, clerics, bioethicists, and legislators) has been poorly informed about the logical basis of the experimental approach and the inherent safety in this orderly, cautious methodology. Misconceptions abound and strong feelings have stood in the way of improvement in understanding. In another context John Kenneth Galbraith, the economist, observed, 'Where reality does not accord with wish our practice is to devise a myth which then serves as a bridge between evidence that cannot be escaped and the belief which is sought.'

The high cost of maintaining the myths which have been devised concerning the subject of clinical experimentation has become substantial and the common good can no longer afford ignorance of this matter. The question, *How* do they know? cannot be avoided; it is a public issue.

An unwitting medical experiment

Doctor John Snow's observations on the occurrence of 286 instances of fatal cholera in districts served by two water companies during the 1854 epidemic in London.

Water company	Fatal attacks of cholera to each of 10 000 houses
Southwark and Vauxhall Co.*	71
Lambeth Co.**	5

* *Source*: water from the Thames at Battersea Fields, about half-a-mile above Vauxhall Bridge, containing 'hairs of animals and numerous substances which had passed through the alimentary canal.'

** *Source*: water works at Thames Ditton 'quite free from the sewage of London.'

THE RANDOMIZED CLINICAL TRIAL

In this book I will focus on a special form of experimentation—the randomized clinical trial—which has been developed to test medical innovations. This alternative to time-honored methods of judging new treatments is the one evaluative strategy which requires the most understanding by the entire community. It cannot be carried out without widespread co-operation.

The details of how doctors perform the technical skills of their craft have little to do with the basic principles of the approach. No specialized medical knowledge is needed to follow the arguments. That is not to say that technological details of experimental maneuvers are not crucially important, but they are usually dwarfed by preceding matters related to straightforward reasoning, to the peculiarly human aspects of experiencing illness, and to the special problems associated with interpreting results in human beings in contrast to other species.

R.A. Fisher's arguments concerning the arrangement of agricultural field trials (1926)

A field trial to test the effectiveness of manure might be conducted as follows:

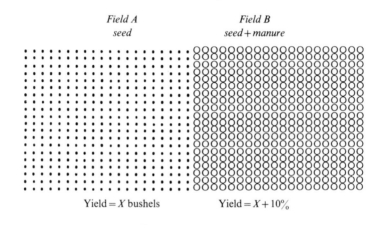

Field A
seed

Field B
seed + manure

Yield = X bushels   Yield = $X + 10\%$

Fisher asked, 'What reason is there to think that, even if no manure had been applied, the acre which received it would not still have given the higher yield?' If the experimenter could say that in twenty years' experience with uniform treatment the difference in favor of Field B had never touched 10 per cent, he could say, 'Either there is something in the treatment or a coincidence has occurred such as does not occur more than once in twenty trials.' The 1 out of 20 likelihood of a difference of this size is indicated very roughly by the experience in twenty successive trials. To determine the 1 in 20 expectation (referred to as the '5 per cent significance level') with any accuracy would require about 500 years' experience. Since the experimenter could not produce a record of 500 years' yields, the direct test of 'significance' was impractical. Nevertheless, Fisher argued, if the experimenter had only ten previous years' records he might still make out a case if he could claim that under uniform treatment the difference in yields had never come *near* to 10 percent excess yield in Field B. From the theory of errors the actual values for the ten years can be used to calculate how frequently a difference of 10 percent might be expected to turn up by chance in ten repeated trials under uniform treatment. Since the only purpose of the ten previous years' experience was to provide an estimate of the expected-by-chance frequency of occurrence of differences of various magnitudes, Fisher proposed a design for obtaining such an estimate from the actual yields in the trial year. He suggested a method of replication in which the test site is partitioned into blocks of equal size:

Each block is further subdivided into a number of plots of smaller size; and within each block (considered separately) the plots are assigned to the contrasting treatments in *random order*:

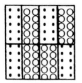

($\bigcirc$ yield) minus ($\bullet$ yield) = block difference

Each block now comprises one replication of the compared treatments. The block differences are used in place of the records of previous years' yields to provide an estimate of deviations. The validity of estimate is now guaranteed by the process of randomization, since each plot has an equal probability of treatment with or without manure. The likelihood of occurrence of difference in yields between the two treatments may now be estimated as before.

Evolution of the randomized trial format

Pioneering development in England   The methodology of the randomized clinical trial is based on principles developed for agricultural research in Britain during the 1920s. R.A. Fisher, a pathfinding biometrist, introduced the concept of random allocation of treatments to subdivided plots of land. He adapted mathematical techniques (developed earlier by Karl Pearson and other workers at the University of London's Laboratory of Biometry, and by William Sealy Gosset who wrote under the pseudonym 'Student') which made it possible to calculate reasonable estimates of variability in yields attributable to chance in field trials.

The Fisherian principles of design and analysis were used in a landmark randomized clinical trial conducted in Britain following World War II to evaluate the streptomycin treatment of tuberculosis. The format of present day trials evolved from this experience and a series of British trials which followed. The influence of A. Bradford Hill, the statistician who played a leading role in the pioneering studies in the UK, and that of Donald Mainland of New York University, has molded the current form.

Methodological standards   Until fairly recently, the mathematical strategies for statistical analysis of experiments received more attention than did the development of principles for examining the underlying conceptual basis of the design of trials involving free-willed doctors and their patients. In recent years, Alvan R. Feinstein of Yale University has examined, in minute detail, the logical 'architecture' of studies conducted under the uniquely distorted conditions encountered in medical settings. From his analyses, those of

David L. Sackett of McMaster University, and of Thomas C. Chalmers of Mount Sinai School of Medicine, a methodological discipline has been developed to help expose the multifold sources of bias which must be taken into account in planning clinical investigations.

Choice between observational and experimental studies in medicine	
Observational studies	*Experimental studies*
Advantages	
1 Practicality 　–greater variety and larger scale of tests of hypotheses, as compared with experiments 　–few ethical objections, since interventions are not imposed by pre-planned design 　–relatively large number of participants can be recruited (especially if only past events are used) 　–duration of study is relatively short (especially when observations are in the form of existing records of past events) 　–relatively inexpensive in time and in personnel (especially when using existing records of past events)	1 Safety 　–relatively few individuals exposed to unpredicted risks in untried interventions 2 Vigor 　–capable of critical tests of limits of applicability 3 Precision 　–theorized causal factor can be defined and limited 　–exposure of test factor under control of experimenter 　–systematic distortions by extraneous factors may be minimized by design 4 Efficiency 　–relatively few observations needed to refute some hypotheses 5 Assumptions 　–random allotment of treatments is assured by design
Disadvantages	
1 Documentation 　–exposure to causal factor less certain 2 Specificity 　–isolating causal factor is difficult 3 Remoteness 　–causal factor and outcome tend to be separated at some distance in time and space 4 Time order 　–direction of relationship between cause and effect less certain 5 Systematic selection 　–availability of patients for treatments 　–allotment of treatments 6 Efficiency of statistical tests 　–lower than experimental designs	1 Impracticality 　–inborn attribute cannot be manipulated 　–predicted risk of intervention is too great 　–long term observation is difficult 　–relatively large number of participants needed to detect small differences 2 Reductionism 　–focus on one independent variable (*The* cause) excludes others from attention 3 Representativeness 　–difficult to recruit a truly random sample from 'universe' 4 Expense 　–relatively great in staff and organizational costs 5 Public acceptance 　–pejorative myths
(Based on arguments of epidemiologist Mervyn Susser)	

Indispensable ordeals

Randomized clinical trials are not without serious limitations. Not the least of these are technical barriers and moral restraints which make it impossible, in some instances, to employ the resolving power of this approach. Other limitations will become obvious as I describe the concepts and operational details in the pages which follow. Nonetheless, this risk-limiting, humanized instrument is the sharpest tool which has been devised for evaluating the limits of applicability of new proposals. Donald S. Fredrickson, former Director of the National Institutes of Health, has pointed out that randomized clinical trials are *indispensable ordeals* in modern medicine.

Even when less powerful testing approaches must be used, the reasoning of the randomized trial lends itself as a guide for setting out specified elements of a clinical problem before we proceed. The analytic process begins by asking, What is the question?—the subject of the next chapter.

'All life is an experiment. It is an endless succession of changes and chances, of risks taken and hunches played, of lions bearded and gauntlets run ...'

Oliver Wendell Holmes

2 Framing the question

In an apocryphal story told by Neil Postman of New York University, an epidemic disease struck a small community and killed many people, but some of the afflicted recovered. The victims lapsed into a deathlike coma and it was hard to know when and, indeed, if they had succumbed. The townspeople worried about burying the 'dead' too soon, and they were hard-pressed for a solution to the dilemma. It was suggested that coffins be well stocked with food and an air vent provided just in case the victim happened to be alive. Although this was expensive, it certainly seemed worth the effort. However, a second proposal was made that was both inexpensive and quite efficient. A twelve-inch stake was to be mounted on the inside of the coffin lid exactly at the level of the heart. When the coffin was closed, all uncertainty would end.

It is of interest that the two solutions were generated by two different questions. The first solution was an answer to the question, How can we make sure that we do not kill people who are alive? The second was a response to the question, How can we be sure that everyone we bury is dead? The point, Postman noted, is that the only answers we get are responses to questions. Although questions that refer to certain assumptions may not be evident, they design the form that our knowledge will take and, thus, determine the course of our actions.

The parable should come to mind as a prelude to the design of clinical studies and before reading the reports of past studies. 'What is the question?' takes precedence over all other considerations.

> 'God is the answer!
> But what is the question?'
> Gertrude Stein

GENUINE QUESTIONS

In order to carry out its directive work effectively, the express question to be addressed in a formal investigation must have the property of authenticity. A question should be considered genuine only if it refers to an hypothesis that can be overturned by defined events. A pseudo-question, on the other hand, is one in which the inferred supposition is at no risk since it cannot be contradicted by any conceivable event. For instance, the query 'Does Galen's treatment (p 2) work?' is a pseudo-question. The claim of infallibility is simply untestable; all treatment failures are ruled out by classifying these unfortunates as 'incurable'.

It is the property of refutability, philosopher Karl Popper has pointed out, that separates scientific questions from those in metaphysics. Moreover, the claims implied in explicit questions are more testable than those in non-specific statements. The former take greater risks of being overthrown and, as a result, are highly productive. What is envisioned is the Galilean interplay of question and experiment: step-by-step challenges of explicit claims with progressive narrowing of the area of uncertainty.

SEARCHING FOR QUESTIONS

Where do the questions come from? Traditionally in medicine they emerge from a background of observation, and I want to turn now to this concept-seeking function of descriptive information. (I will postpone a discussion of other aspects of observation, e.g. sense perception, observer behavior, and measurement until Chapters 6 and 7, which deal with outcome observations in experimental trials.)

Classification of question-seeking observations

Claude Bernard recognized two levels of observation:

'... A spontaneous or passive observation which the physician makes by chance and without being led to it by any preconceived idea ... [secondly] an active observation ... made with a preconceived idea, with intention to verify the accuracy of a mental conception.'

Although the dichotomy is only relative (since the notion of unprejudiced observation is a myth), the classification is, nonetheless, very useful. It deserves a close look. Notice that the distinction between 'passive' and 'active' is made on the basis of the mind-set of the observer.

'Passive' observation A 'passive' observation is made by chance in the sense that it is unexpected according to the (unspoken) prevailing theory about the state of the world. The event or circumstance seems novel because

it was unpredicted and the observation may be considered 'passive' because the viewer did not prepare the physical act of perception with the mental acts of *new* theory formulation and forecast.

'Active' observation   By contrast, the 'active' observation is made after some mental work has been performed. The point here is that a second-level observation is carried out in a newly defined framework of meaning specified in advance by the preconceived idea.

The hierarchal distinction is quite important because it takes notice of a progression in the pre-experimental screening of question-seeking observations. Since there is no end to the number of observables, we need to pick out the observations that are worth further exploration. The move from noting unpredicted incidents to the focus on prediction-confirmed events is just such a culling action; it narrows the search for challenging questions.

An epidemic of blindness

Concrete examples of the two levels of observation took place in 1949 and 1951 when an unexplained epidemic of blindness—retrolental fibroplasia, or RLF—affecting prematurely-born infants, raged throughout the United States and, to a lesser extent, in other countries throughout the world (see Appendix A for a history of RLF).

Boston survey   The experience with RLF in several US cities was surveyed in 1949 by V. Everett Kinsey and Leona Zacharias of Boston's Eye and Ear Infirmary, in the hope that some cause might be identified to account for the sudden increase of the previously rare disorder. Forty-seven factors relating to mothers and infants delivered in Boston between the years 1938 and 1948 were examined and these (for example, complications of pregnancy, delivery, and the newborn period; treatments administered to mother and baby; and so forth) were correlated with the occurrence of RLF.

The investigators had two goals in mind: to enumerate the conditions and treatments experienced by children affected and unaffected by RLF and to compare the trends of factors and outcomes over an interval before and after the sharp rise in frequency of RLF. But they had no single and *specific* hypothesis in mind. (The analytic procedure used has been termed 'data-dredging'; data obtained in the past are disinterred, as with a dredge, to see what turns up.)

On completion of the survey, the observers discovered associations between increased RLF-blindness in premature infants and treatment with iron salts, the administration of water-miscible vitamins, and liberal use of oxygen therapy. Curves demonstrating time trends of the unpredicted correlations led the Boston authors to report that 'correlation between the rise

'Passive' associations in a Boston survey

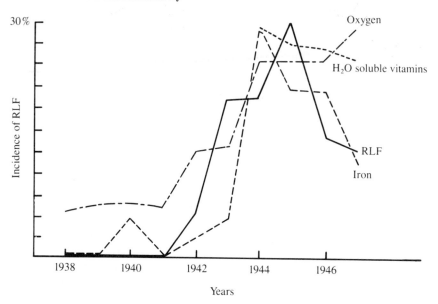

Occurrence of RLF-blindness and the administration of three treatments to premature infants in a Boston nursery from 1938 to 1947. The vertical axis indicates the occurrence of RLF (range 0–30 per cent), the duration of oxygen treatment (range 0–15 days), drops of water-miscible vitamins (range 0–400 drops), and grains of iron sulfate (range 0–60 grains). The study population consisted of 53 RLF-blind and 298 sighted children born some years before the study began. (Redrawn from the data of Kinsey and Zacharias)

in incidence and [treatments] was less striking for oxygen than for water-miscible vitamin preparations and for iron.'

Rarity, interest and surprise   Before going on, it would be worth pausing for a moment to consider the concepts of rarity, interest, and surprise as they relate to observations of events in medicine.

For example, the Boston analysts were quite justified in regarding the associations found in their survey as rarities: simple inspection of the distribution of the frequencies is convincing. (Even without statistical arithmetic, it is safe to say that co-events like these would be expected to occur rarely by chance alone.) Moreover, the associations were unquestionably interesting: the analysts (and the baffled medical community) were very much interested in the findings of the survey. What remains to be examined is the matter of surprise: Were the results surprising?

The requirements for justified astonishment were set out many years ago by mathematician Warren Weaver. He argued that an event should not be considered surprising merely because it is rare (i.e. the probability of occurrence is small in an *absolute sense*), but rather because its probability is quite small as compared with the probabilities of other possible alternatives.

In the Boston survey, a large number of 'alternative' correlates were examined (when the survey was undertaken, there was no theory concerning a mechanism of action of these factors). Thus, the likelihood of concurrence of any one of these forty-odd variants with RLF, simply as a meaningless coincidence, was of the same low order of probability as a fortuitous association with iron salts, vitamins, and oxygen. It was reasonable to conclude that the associations observed in this survey were rare and quite interesting. But they were *not* surprising. In fact, if the dredging process had continued long enough, other associations would have been found, as guaranteed by the definition of improbable events.

The fundamental distinction between impossible events and improbable events is that the former cannot occur and the latter *must* occur if the observations continue indefinitely. (Following the Boston survey, other searches turned up haphazard correlations between the occurrence of RLF and cow's milk feedings, blood transfusions, low fluid intake, and rapid cessation of oxygen treatment.)

This, then, is the underlying weakness of 'passive' observations: incredibly rare events are occurring all around us; if we single out those which have already occurred because they are of interest to us, we cannot, with any confidence, attribute 'significance' or 'meaning' to their occurrence. We have no right to be surprised. And this is the basis for a fundamental tenet of the scientific method: hypotheses to be tested must be formulated before examining the data that are to be used to test them.

Melbourne prediction   How does the situation differ in the case of 'active' observations? Here the relationship between the possible alternatives is changed by declaring the outcome-of-interest *before* examining the outcome-in-fact.

For example, in 1951, an Australian physician, Kate Campbell, heard a rumor that RLF frequency increased in Britain when oxygen use was liberalized (after inception of the National Health Service made increased funds available for the purchase of medical equipment). She proceeded to examine the experience of babies in three Melbourne hospitals with the preconceived idea that RLF occurrence might be related to the use of oxygen. And she found that the disorder was most frequent in the institution which used oxygen freely.

The association found by this 'active' observation was more credible than the correlations noted earlier in Boston. Note, however, that the improved quality of the new evidence was not based on the numbers of babies in-

RLF in Melbourne

Years	Free use of oxygen[a] (*Institution I*)		Conservative use of oxygen[b] (*Institutions II and III*)	
1948–50	No. of Infants 123	No. with RLF 23	No. of Infants 58	No. with RLF 4
RLF%	19%		7%	

a. In Institution I oxygen was piped into the ward and was given in an oxygen cot: the percentage of oxygen ranged between 40 and 60 per cent. Oxygen was given before symptoms appeared as well as during periods of obvious need (blue spells).
b Institutions II and III oxygen was administered sparingly (by a catheter placed in the nose or by a funnel placed over the face, sometimes by tent or closed cot).
(Taken from the observations of Campbell)

volved in the two sets of observations nor on any calculation of the comparative rarity-by-chance of the Boston and Melbourne experiences. Both sets of observations were certainly of considerable interest. But the distinctive qualities of the 'active' observation were: 1) the Melbourne thesis satisfied Popper's requirement—it risked failure by predicting a high frequency of RLF only in hospitals using oxygen liberally, and 2) it satisfied Weaver's requirement for surprise—the association was unusual as *compared with all other associations considered together.*

It is as if I declare that only a bridge hand of thirteen spades interests me and lump together all other hands as imperfect. The probability of drawing any specified bridge hand on a single deal is vanishingly small (1 divided by 635 013 559 600) and none are surprising since each one of the thousands of millions of possibilities is equally rare. My proclaimed hand becomes surprising only when I compare it with the sum of the probabilities of the alternatives (the likelihood of receiving an imperfect hand approaches certainty). Moreover, if I am dealt a hand of thirteen spades, I may become

---

A misunderstanding about chance

Horace C. Levinson, the mathematician, illustrated a common misunderstanding about *a priori* probability by relating the story of an embattled sailor who put his head through the first hole made in the side of his ship by an enemy cannon ball. The man reasoned that it was highly improbable that another ball would come through the same hole.

Although the sailor was correct in believing it was highly unlikely that two balls would hit the ship at the same spot, he was entirely mistaken in his belief that after the first strike the likelihood of an identical repeat is smaller than the chance it would hit any other spot *designated in advance.* Before the engagement began, the betting odds were huge against two balls landing on the same spot, but once half the 'miracle' had been accomplished, the betting odds were immediately reduced to the odds that any indicated point would be safe.

suspicious about the dealing process or the dealer, but the happening is invested with considerably more 'meaning' if I declare my suspicion *before* the deal. Again, the improbability of the event as reckoned before its occurrence is the same in both instances, but rarity of the hand is not as important as the level of observation.

The mere fact that a probability is low should not in itself lead to amazement. I am not justified in declaring, 'This event *must* have some meaning because the probability of occurrence by pure chance is incredibly remote—surely nothing as improbable as this could ever occur.' An evening of bridge is convincing evidence that the occurrence of events of fantastically small probabilities is, in fact, inevitable.

DATA-DREDGING PROCEDURES

Quite often in medicine, we are faced with baffling disorders or phenomena and we are forced to begin the search for meaning with very weak questions (as in the 1949 survey: What can account for the rise in RLF?). In the absence of any reasonable specific theory, it is entirely reasonable to undertake an epidemiologic survey of unplanned events which have already occurred, but it is prudent to take some precautions.

The problem has been likened, by economists Hanan C. Selvin and Alan Stuart, to a hunter stalking an unknown quarry through an unfamiliar landscape with an arsenal of complex weapons. The evocative names they have given to two of several data-dredging procedures in survey analysis are 'fishing' and 'hunting'.

'Fishing'

When pre-search questions are vague, the principal motive for embarking on a survey is to provide the observational material from which a precise theory may be formed. This process of angling for a model is quite literally a 'fishing expedition', using the observed data to choose which of a number of candidate determinants to include in an explanatory thesis.

Once a 'fish' is caught, the survey analyst must have a different body of data to evaluate the explanatory model developed in the first search. This need not involve a new set of observations if the initial collection was divided (with suitable precautions to insure that the sub-sets are not too dissimilar) into two parts for just this purpose.

For example, the Boston survey might have employed this 'double-pond' approach by using half of the observations for 'fishing'. When the three 'fish' (iron, vitamins, and oxygen) were landed, the remaining half of the experience could have been used to make 'active' observations about the associations in the unexamined pool of information held in reserve.

'Hunting'

'Fishing' uses a limited number of candidate variables, but 'hunting' involves no restrictions. The data are widely probed for information in the area of interest. The practice can take many forms. Basically it involves searching through a body of data and examining many relations in order to find rare co-occurrences. Or one can examine a single hypothesis seeking confirmations in many different bodies of data.

The practice leads to a pernicious problem when only 'significant' results are published, but I will return to this in a later chapter. Suffice it to say here that 'hunting' offers the maximum scope for the data stalker since there are no ground rules.

A 'hunting accident' The history of medicine is rich with stories of 'hunting accidents'. One such event occurred in 1949 when the results of treating 179 newborn infants with exchange transfusion were examined. This technique

A 'hunting accident'

Sex of blood donor and survival of babies* after exchange transfusion

Sex of blood donor	Outcome of exchange transfusion		
	No. treated	*No. survived*	*Per cent survived*
Male	137	110	*80%***
Female	42	42	*100%***

* Newborn infants suffering from anemia and jaundice (erythroblastosis fetalis).
** These proportions were processed with statistical arithmetic and the difference was declared 'significant'; that is, the likelihood of obtaining a similar difference in survival by chance alone is less than 1 in 100 repeated trials involving comparable numbers of patients.
(Taken from the data of F.H. Allen, Jr. and others)

of replacing blood had been introduced the year before as a method for preventing death and brain damage in infants who were born with erythroblastosis fetalis, a severe form of anemia and jaundice caused by Rh-blood-group incompatability between mother and fetus. The analysts wrote that they were surprised to note that although mortality was over 15 per cent in the whole group, there were no deaths in a group of 42 babies who happened to receive blood from female blood donors exclusively.

The unexpected observation prompted a searching analysis in the *same* collection of data (10 other state-of-the-mother-and-infant variables were examined) and the authors concluded that 'it appears certain that exchange transfusion using blood from a female donor is the treatment of choice for babies with erythroblastosis fetalis. In the past two months we have given this type of blood by exchange transfusion to 13 babies with erythroblastosis fetalis. All have recovered.' A report of the female-donor benefit appeared as the lead article in a highly-regarded medical journal and attracted widespread interest. However, the authors had wisely advised that others examine their own experiences for evidence of a similar beneficial effect. It was quickly found that the hopeful results could not be duplicated in subsequent studies.

PROBLEMS INDUCED BY VARIABILITY

I have noted that questions and bold new theories in medicine arise from a number of sources. Informal, yet accurate, on-going personal observations of events by practising physicians (case studies) have been fundamental to progress in the past and they remain indispensable as a source of original hypotheses. But the shift of emphasis from the individual patient to groups of patients (populations) as the unit of study reflects a change in thinking about causality in medicine.

A simple view of causal relationships, a single cause resulting in a single effect, is gradually being replaced by a concept of multiple causes and variable consequences.

Variation in medical events

The change in outlook emphasizes the difference between the type of uniformity that can be contrived in the laboratory or seen in repetitions of phenomena that give the same result over and over (such as the time required for a ball to fall from a fixed height) and the case to case irregularity that characterizes medical incidents (for example, the course of illness with or without treatment). Invariable outcomes, such as death or disability, are rare, and infallible treatments are virtually non-existent in medicine.

It is the variability in clinical events that leads to the need for *collections* of observations to generate explicit (number-specific) questions and the need for some method of untangling the strands in a web of relationships so the questions can be tested rigorously.

Oxygen and RLF   Many of the problems of variability were encountered during the early attempts to explain the rise of RLF. I said that the preconceived Melbourne idea concerning a causal relationship between oxygen treatment and RLF received substantial support from the observations in compared hospitals (p 18). Now I must point out the weakness in that evidence.

First, the majority of infants who received liberal oxygen treatment did not develop RLF; only one-fifth of the babies so treated were affected. Clearly, other risk determinants exerted a considerable influence on outcome. And there was no assurance that these unfavorable factors were distributed equally among the groups of babies in the surveyed hospitals.

Secondly, the prediction concerning an assoociation between treatment and outcome failed to specify *in advance* the size of difference in RLF

Francis Galton's contribution to the study of cause and effect

Francis Galton's introduction of the idea of correlation in 1889 opened the way to a deeper study of the problems of cause and effect. Up to that time, only simple causal relations could be described in quantitative terms. His concept provided a means for mathematical analysis of multiple causes: 'the degree of relationship, or of partial causality, between the different variables of our ever-changing universe' could be represented by a system of numbers.

Galton began by comparing the size of two generations of seeds from cress plants (the size of seeds sown and the size of seeds produced by their progeny). He attempted to formalize the associations by sorting the mother seeds into five size categories and similarly ranking daughter seeds produced in each of the seeds-sown categories. Thirty groups (5 sown and 25 produced; each size grade in small, round containers) were set out in a tabular array:

The sixth vertical column of Galton's 'table' (labeled 'sizes of the seeds sown') ranked the five containers of parent seed by size (from the largest '$+2°$' to the smallest '$-2°$'); each of the horizontal rows displayed the seeds of progeny in similar rank order. The array was covered with a sheet of glass and a series of contour lines were drawn connecting seed ranks of similar size (Galton termed these 'isograms'; the lines are smudged and almost obliterated).

The rough observations contained the germ of an idea for measuring the intensity of resemblance between characteristics exhibiting a range of variability due to 'different and equally probable combinations of a multitude of small independent causes.' Galton went on to develop a mathematical approach to associations between many kinds of measurements; the dimensions were expressed in statistical terms and relationships were summarized as coefficients of correlation. His insight revolutionized the study of natural phenomena.

occurrence that would be accepted as decisive. Since the range of possible differences was large in this highly variable disorder (a wide range of occurrence was reported in groups of babies who were presumed to be treated uniformly, see p 35), a single confirmation of the numberless prediction was not entirely convincing.

Discordances between an isolated 'cause' and an isolated effect in medicine
(For Example: Supplemental Oxygen and RLF)

'Cause' and effect associations	*The 'cause' is necessary*	*The 'cause' is sufficient*
A	+	+
B	+	−
C	−	+
D	−	−

A. The 'cause' is necessary and it is sufficient to result in the effect. Such a straightforward relationship is referred to as *deterministic* causality. For example, if exposure to supplemental oxygen and nothing but such exposure was needed to cause RLF, it would be logical to consider this agent as the sole necessary and sufficient cause of RLF. In late 1954 when such a relationship was 'established', research activities into matters related to the disorder virtually ceased. Over the next 20 years, it slowly became evident that this simplistic causal model was inadequate.

B. The 'cause' is necessary but it is not sufficient to result in the effect. Here there is a producer-product relationship, and the term *probabilistic* (nondeterministic) causality may be applied. Early in the investigation of the association between supplemental oxygen and RLF, it was noted that exposure to supplemental oxygen did not result in RLF in all newborn infants. An additional factor, immature development of the blood vessels of the eye, was found to be a necessary determinant. Moreover, only a minority of immaturely developed infants exposed to the treatment developed RLF. Slowly it was realized that there must be other determinants not yet identified.

C. The 'cause' is not necessary but it is sufficient to result in the effect. The association is referred to as *correlation* (the purported 'cause' and the effect tend to be present or absent together); the association may not involve causality at all. For instance, it became evident that RLF occurred in a few infants who had never been exposed to supplemental oxygen. This supported the suspicion that there were multiple causes of RLF—or that the incompletely developed eye could be adversely influenced by the oxygen (21 per cent) in atmospheric air.

D. The 'cause' is neither necessary nor is it sufficient to result in the effect. For instance, RLF was found in some stillborn infants. Here the mechanism appeared to be related to severe oxygen *lack*. Recently there has been reason to suspect that exposure to oxygen after birth may be only a contributory determinant; the causal role may have been exaggerated when the gas was administered in high concentrations for prolonged periods of time (in the years before 1955).

(Adapted from Mervyn Susser's arguments)

The numerical method and the idea of formal comparisons in medicine

The concept of formal enumeration in medicine had its origin in the London Bills of Mortality which were kept regularly beginning with publication of the bill dated December 29, 1603. (Earlier Bills, which furnished the number of deaths caused by the plague compared with all other fatal sickness, began in 1532, but these appeared only sporadically.) The London Bills described medical events in the parishes; they were published on the Thursday before Christmas Day. In the year 1665, London experienced the last of many epidemics of plague:

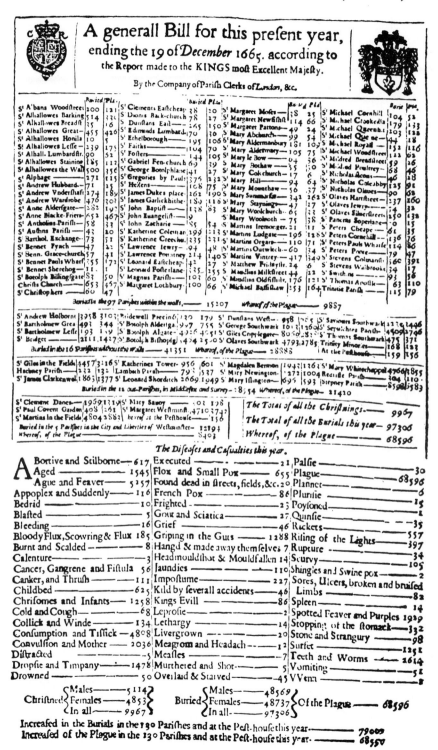

A generall Bill for this present year, ending the 19 of *December* 1665. according to the Report made to the KINGS most Excellent Majesty.

By the Company of Parish Clerks of *London*, &c.

For many years, the death rolls were used merely to warn the sovereign of the need to move to clean air. Major Greenwood, the British statistician, reviewed this period in the history of medical statistics. He came upon some novel questions for the Bills to answer in the papers and correspondence of a sceptical physician, William Petty:

'Whether of 1000 patients to the best physicians, aged of any decade, there do not die as many as out of the inhabitants of places where there dwell no physicians. Whether of 100 sick of acute diseases who use physicians, as many die and in misery, as where no art is used, or only chance.'

Although these particular analyses were never carried out, the seed of the idea of formal comparisons was planted. Out of the casual correspondence between Petty and his friend, John Graunt, in the mid 17th Century, a new method of scientific investigation germinated and grew slowly.

It became important to know if the observed discrepancy in RLF risk was reproducible. Experiences in other parts of the world were quickly examined but the issues remained unsettled. Some observers found an increased risk with oxygen treatment, others found no association; one found a decreased risk (the early changes of RLF improved when infants were placed in oxygen-enriched incubators), and RLF occurred in some babies who were never treated with oxygen.

The descriptive studies served to sharpen the questions that needed to be asked about oxygen treatment, such as: What gas concentration and duration of treatment is used? What groups of premature infants are susceptible? What specific eye changes are diagnostic of RLF? What range of difference in risk of RLF is expected in treated and non-treated groups? But a firm link between cause and effect was not established by the observational methods.

NUMERICAL APPROACH TO VARIABILITY

The complexities introduced by variability in illness outcomes were recognized by William Petty, a 17th century English physician, who proposed that groups of patients be compared in order to distinguish between 'art' and 'chance'. Ironically, this fertile idea grew more rapidly in other fields of biology than in medicine.

I have already noted that the class of problems in which exact outcomes are not predictable was recognized by experimenters in agriculture. The techniques of numerical comparison permitted them to work with the evidence as they found it and to measure an effect against the background of fluctuations. They did not try to idealize an experiment, and, instead, accepted the reality of variability 'caused' by multiple influences.

The move from descriptive study to a statistical kind of experimentation which made it possible to approach the problem of uncontrollable confounding factors in a real-world setting was a major step in the biological sciences. Mathematician and philosopher Jacob Bronowski said of this revolutionary shift to statistical methodology: 'It replaces the concept of *inevitible effect* by that of the *probable trend*.' (It is interesting that when the investigation of physical phenomena reached subatomic dimensions, physicists encountered uncertainties of the kind so familiar in biology. For guidance, they employed the statistical outlook which had already been developed in biological research.)

Statistical reasoning

A central question needs to be considered when statistical reasoning is used in human experimentation: How do we decide whether or not a pattern of observed events (or measurements) is to be attributed to chance (random occurrences) or to systematic influences (that is, to a planned intervention or to unplanned forces that we classify as bias)?

It is very important to understand that our ability to nullify biasing influences rests entirely on precautions taken in the design of an experimental plan. (Most of the space in this book will be taken up with discussions of the control of bias). Statistical methods do not offer a formula to distinguish between planned and unplanned *systematic* influences. On the other hand, numerical analysis provides a tool that allows us (with reasonable assurance) to differentiate random from non-random patterns of outcome.

Forecasting in gambling   It is useful to compare the happenings we encounter in medicine with the events in games of chance. For the reasoning of the gambler (not devil-may-care as he would have us believe) leads the way to a practical approach to the problems which bedevil physicians.

In the simple game of 'heads or tails', for example, the results in successive tosses of a coin may be thought of as a series. The separate outcomes (like the single events in medicine) seem to occur erratically when we confine our attention to a few tosses at a time. But when the results in a long succession are examined, a pattern emerges. Finally the regularities of the workings of chance are quite distinct.

In a game involving hundreds of throws of a coin, the proportion of 'heads' or 'tails' is likely to be very close to one-half. And, in a very large experience, runs of successive 'heads' and of 'tails' also approach fixed proportions of the total. The point here is that in examining a long series of events (both in coin tossing and in medicine) order gradually emerges out of disorder.

Although there are enormous differences between the complex events in medicine and the straightforward occurrences in coin tossing, both provide the same kind of information needed to make predictions about repeated series of similar observations. However, a gambler has the very practical advantage of being able to calculate theoretical probabilities of outcomes *before* making any real world observations.

Several reasonable assumptions are made: 1. the physical forces that may influence the outcome of each toss operate haphazardly—they do not align themselves in favor of either 'heads' or 'tails'; 2. since the coin has no memory, the outcome of each toss is not influenced by preceding results; and 3. all of the possible and equally likely outcomes are obvious by inspecting the coin. Once these are accepted, the probabilities of various outcomes that will be approached in an up-coming game can be computed with equations based on the laws of chance.

If the results in a number of games do not agree with those predicted by theory, the gambler may be led to frame a new hypothesis, one which specifies the expected behavior of the unusual coin in hand.

Forecasting in medicine The doctor is unable to calculate the 'expected' proportions of outcomes in advance; the phrase 'all possible and equally likely events', so obvious by looking at a coin, has no clear meaning in complex problems. In medicine we are obliged to appeal to experience for statistical probabilities.

The variation, for example, in the occurrence of blindness begins to approach a fixed proportion in a long series of observations of infants treated with oxygen. After this information is in hand, we can make predictions with the same confidence as in a game of coin-tossing (or in weather forecasts, insurance risks, highway-accident projections ... and predictions made about many events in the natural world about which we have little or no precise 'causal' knowledge). The regularities in the aggregate make it possible to make inferences from what John Venn, the probability theorist, called 'proportional propositions'.

Uncomfortable as it is to dwell on the analogy, the resemblance between the gambler and the physician cannot be denied. Both must frame their questions about the state of the world in numerical terms. The gambler's hope for 'doctored' coins that will defy *a priori* calculations of outcome are exactly like the hopes of physicians for favorable treatments. Both dream of winning by consistently upsetting usual outcome probabilities, but both are forced to test their fantasies in real world experiments.

MEANINGFUL QUESTIONS

Now that I have argued for asking number-specific questions when planning clinical trials (and I will develop the details of this issue in Chapter 9), I must emphasize that reality imposes an additional demand. It must not be forgotten that medical events, unlike those encountered in the casino or in the laboratory, are complex social phenomena with wide ramifications.

Research questions, it has been said, are like blinkers on a horse; they resist distraction, but they limit the possibilities of perception by removing the context in which meaning is embedded. The horse must remember to turn his head from time to time.

The questions asked in human experiments cannot be framed in a vacuum; there must be some kind of value judgment—a community consensus about 'meaning'—that validates the inquiries. For example, clinical trials are undertaken to increase the store of medical knowledge and to provide practical information that can be applied in the practice of medicine. The relative emphasis given to the two objectives in a specific trial requires a decision heavily influenced by the public interest.

Step-by-step questions

The growth of applied knowledge in medicine can be envisaged as a continuous process in which each cycle begins with good questions and ends with better questions. I can appreciate how disconcerting it is to read these words about a body of knowledge in which we all have a vested interest, a system of information that is concerned with our well-being and our lives. Common sense demands a search for better *answers*. But a little reflection should make it obvious that the 'answers' in bedside medicine are ephemeral. (The 'half-life' of medical knowledge is constantly shrinking.) In the presence of uncertainties, it is the questions, as illustrated in the parable at the beginning of this chapter, that are doing their work. *They* determine the course of our actions.

> 'We have learned the answers, all the answers:
> It is the question that we do not know.'
> Archibald MacLeish

3 Representative patients

Explanatory and pragmatic goals in clinical trials are so intertwined that attempts to make a clear separation between them seem contrived. And yet, as I have noted, a public-value-guided choice to emphasize one or the other of the two aims must be made. They cannot be pursued with equal vigor in a single trial. French biostatistician Daniel Schwartz and his co-workers have argued that a choice between the two purposes must be taken into account at every stage in the design of a comparative trial and in analysis of results. For example, a purely explanatory trial is conducted with idealized patients under restricted conditions in an effort to demonstrate specifically predicted biologic effects of a new treatment. The pragmatic trial seeks to assess the practical value of a new treatment when given to a wide range of patients in usual medical settings. In this book I have focused on trial formats which emphasize the latter approach.

Pragmatic trials are carried out in the hope that results will provide a reliable guide for future treatment policy. But such generalization requires a leap that must not be undertaken lightly. I have indicated that forecasting in medicine requires an appeal to experience. Now we need to examine an important requirement of experience used to predict results that doctors can expect when they prescribe for their patients. The experience must be representative.

RANDOM SAMPLING MODEL

The idealized model for establishing the ground rules that enable us to make inferences about unexamined cases comes from direct experiments in random sampling. The underlying idea is that we can obtain information about the whole by examining only a part. The statistical reasoning is the same as that used for forecasting outcomes in games of chance. In the classic example, a jar is filled with black and white marbles in some undisclosed ratio and we remove a sample set. From the proportions observed in the sample, we make statements about the actual distribution in the jar (that is, the ranges within which the proportions are expected to lie); and we assign a graded quantity of belief to these assertions.

Assumptions

The entire operation hinges on the matter of representative sampling. Thus, we need some assurances before a test set of marbles is removed. We must assume that the marbles do not have inherent characteristics, such as 'stickiness', differential weights, and internal 'motors'; and that they cannot be maneuvered by external forces, such as 'magnetism' which would favor systematic aggregation. We must also be assured that there is an unequivocal distinction between black and white marbles (no grays). And the jar must be well stirred to assure random scattering before a sample is removed.

The word 'random'   The connotations of the word 'random' deserve some attention here. The term frequently implies dynamic movement or occurrence that takes place without aim, purpose, or fixed principle. Another connotation—at liberty and free from restraint or control—is also relevant in the present context. The scientific meaning of 'random distribution' was made clear by Venn who pointed to the arrangement of drops of rain in a shower. 'No one can guess', he said, 'where a drop will fall at any one instant, but we know that if we put out a sheet of paper, it will gradually become uniformly spotted all over. And equal areas on the paper will gradually tend to be struck equally often.'

From sample observation to population estimate

If the pre-sampling assumptions are reasonable, batch testing may proceed with confidence. The proportion observed in a random sample will provide a calculable estimate of the true ratio of black and white marbles in the jar which is termed the 'target population', 'parent population', or 'population of interest'. Notice that this population is related only vaguely to the 'universe' of marbles which exists outside of the jar.

GROUPS OF PATIENTS

The ideas that lie behind the simple marble-sampling model should be kept in mind when considering the recruitment of a group of patients who will serve as representatives in a planned clinical study, but it is important from the outset to recognize the limitations of the analogy as we enter the complicated real world. The inherent characteristics of patients which influence their systematic choices of physicians and hospitals, their susceptibility to 'magnetic' external forces represented by the medical system, the blurred distinctions between categories of patients, and their resistance to thorough 'stirring' virtually guarantee sampling difficulties. The qualities that distin-

ESTIMATION OF PROPORTIONS IN A PARENT POPULATION
SAMPLING
Empirical Results* versus Computation** of the Binomial Probability Distribution

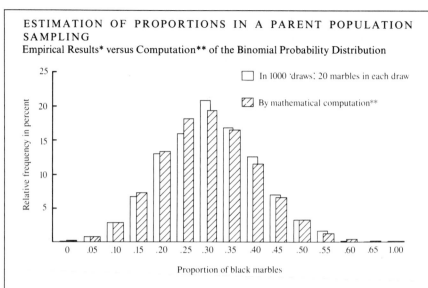

Proportion of black marbles

* Frequency of occurrence (in per cent) of 20-marble samples with specified proportions of black marbles.

** Expansion of the binomial formula $(p+q)^{20}$
where $p = 0.3$ = the proportion of black marbles in the jar,
    $q = 0.7$ = the proportion of white marbles in the jar, and the exponent[20] is the number of marbles in each sample drawn from the jar.
In the sampling experiment conducted by Mainland, 300 black marbles and 700 white marbles were placed in a jar, the contents thoroughly mixed, 20 marbles were drawn, the result noted, and the marbles returned to the jar. The sampling procedure was continued until 1000 samples of 20 were obtained. The frequency distribution of proportions of black marbles obtained by the empirical approach is very close to the values obtained by mathematical computation. In this example, samples which contained fewer than 10 per cent black marbles (zero or one black marble in twenty), and more than 55 per cent (more than 11 black marbles in twenty) occurred rarely; less than 5 per cent of the samples fell into these extreme tails of a normal distribution.
    An estimate of the sampling 'error' may be expressed by the formula:

$$\text{S.D.} = \sqrt{\frac{p \times q}{n}}$$

where S.D. = the standard deviation (in some contexts it is termed, the standard error) of
    a percentage of a dichotomous (either/or) property,
    p = the percentage of black marbles observed in the sample
    q = the percentage of white marbles in the sample
    n = the number of marbles in the sample
The percentages in the parent population are estimated within given 'confidence limits'. In a hypothetical example, we draw a single sample of 20 marbles from the jar of 300 black and 700 white marbles, and count 5 black marbles (25 per cent) in the set, thus

$$\text{S.D.} = \sqrt{\frac{25\% \times 75\%}{20}} = 9.7\%$$

In repeated samples of 20 drawn from the jar, we expect that the percentage of black marbles will lie within $p + 2$ S.D. and $p - 2$ S.D. (25 per cent ± 19.4 per cent), and that values will be found outside these limits about once in twenty draws. Thus, we estimate that the percentage of black marbles in the jar (as judged by this hypothetical single draw) lies somewhere between 5.6 per cent and 44.4 per cent; and we expect to be wrong about 5 per cent of the time. If we increase the sample size tenfold to 200 marbles, the range of the 'confidence limits' is reduced by a factor of 3 (now 25 per cent $\pm$ 6.1 per cent estimates that the percentage in the jar lies between 18.9 per cent and 31.1 per cent; and in this hypothetical instance the percentage in the jar, 30 per cent, lies within the range estimated by the single sample draw of 200 marbles).

guish *all* groups of patients are far removed from the connotation 'at liberty and free from restraint or control.'

Haphazard sampling in medicine

There is widespread belief in a disturbing misconception that if the source of the patients is not known, the sample is a random one. The misunderstanding stems from failure to make a distinction between everyday use of the word 'random', which leans toward the idea of 'without aim, purpose, or fixed principle,' and the use by statisticians. The latter are concerned with the process of random sampling in a precise technical sense in order to fulfill the assumptions of probability theory. The term 'probability samples' is sometimes used by statisticians to avoid confusion.

Edmond A. Murphy of Johns Hopkins University has pointed out that it is not an uncommon practice when attempting to establish 'normal values' of blood constituents, to collect specimens from groups of people in blood banks, from technicians working in a laboratory, or from people walking down a hospital corridor. A sample of this kind is not, as investigators may imagine, a random sample of the population. It is, he emphasized, merely a haphazard one. If the conclusions about 'normal values' are to be extended to a wide population, say the entire country, we must go to some lengths to satisfy the probability sampling requirement that each person in the entire population is *equally likely* to be chosen for the sample. In a formal study, sampling difficulties should be recognized and shortcomings should be reported.

Target population

To deal with the problem of recruiting representative patients, we are first obliged to define the target population: To whom are the results of the study meant to apply? The answer, which spells out the *external relevance* of the investigation, is usually more parochial than hoped for. Limitations are imposed because of the way in which patients aggregate in various parts of the medical system.

'Available' patients   For example, studies are conducted most commonly in groups of patients chosen from those who are 'available'; they turn up in hospitals, out-patient departments, and doctors' offices. Referral patterns

Some biases in specifying and selecting the study sample

Admission rate (Berkson) bias

    If hospitalization rates differ for different exposure/disease groups, the relation between exposure and disease will become distorted in hospital-based studies.

Centripetal bias

    The reputations of certain physicians and medical institutions cause individuals with specific disorders or exposures to gravitate toward them.

Detection signal (unmasking) bias

    An innocent factor may become suspect if it causes a sign or symptom which sets off an intensified search for the disease.

Diagnostic access bias

    Individuals differ in their geographic, temporal, and economic access to the diagnostic procedures which label them as having a given disease.

Diagnostic suspicion bias

    A knowledge of the subject's prior exposure to a putative cause (ethnicity, taking a certain drug, having a second disorder, being exposed in an epidemic) may influence both the intensity and the outcome of the diagnostic process.

Diagnostic vogue bias

    The same illness may receive different diagnostic labels at different points in space or time.

Membership bias

    Membership in a group (the employed, joggers, etc.) may imply a degree of health which differs systematically from that of the general population.

Non-contemporaneous controls bias

    Secular changes in definitions, exposures, diagnoses, diseases, and treatments may render non-contemporaneous controls non-comparable.

Non-respondent bias

    Non-respondents (or 'late-comers') from a specified sample may exhibit exposures or outcomes which differ from those of respondents (or 'early-comers').

Popularity bias

    The admission of patients to some doctors' practices, medical institutions, or procedures (surgery, autopsy) is influenced by the interest stirred up by the presenting condition and its possible causes.

Prevalence-incidence (Neyman) bias

    A late look at those exposed (or affected) early will miss fatal or other short episodes, plus mild or 'silent' cases and cases in which evidence of exposure disappears with disease onset.

Previous opinion bias

    The tactics and results of a previous diagnostic process on a patient, if known, may effect the tactics and results of a subsequent diagnostic process on the same patient.

Procedure selection bias

    Certain clinical procedures may be preferentially offered to those who are poor risks. (Selection of patients for 'medical' vs 'surgical' therapy.)

Referral filter bias

    As a group of ill are referred from primary to secondary to tertiary care facilities, the concentration of rare causes, multiple diagnoses, and 'hopeless cases' may increase.

Unacceptable disease bias

    When disorders are socially unacceptable (V.D., suicide, insanity) they tend to be under-reported.

Volunteer bias

    Volunteers or 'early comers' from a specified sample may exhibit exposures or outcomes (they tend to be healthier) which differ from those of non-volunteers or 'late-comers'.

(Described by Sackett)

of physicians, special interests in particular hospitals, admission practices (when hospitals are crowded, only the most severe cases of a particular disease are admitted and when many beds are free, milder cases may be admitted also), and the hierarchical organization of hospitals (into primary, secondary, and tertiary care centers of increasing specialization) all tend to bring about an irreproducible sorting of patients. As a result, the characteristics of hospital patients may vary widely from institution to institution. Generalizations based on observations in hospitalized groups are notoriously untrustworthy. In one study, hospitalized patients with respiratory diseases had arthritis complaints twice as often as those not affected with respiratory difficulties. This 'increased risk of arthritis' was not observed in comparable patients who were not in hospitals. The spurious association is an example of what is called 'Berkson's Bias', one of a long list of selection biases collected by Sackett.

Dissimilar babies　The 1949 survey of the occurrence of RLF among infants reared in hospitals throughout the United States (p 16) is another example of the difficulties in obtaining groups of 'typical' patients for formal study. As I have said, the occurrence of blindness and treatment practices varied considerably from hospital to hospital and in the same hospital over time. This confusion was further compounded by dissimilarities in the at-risk populations. In addition to the relatively small numbers of observations reported by some of the hospitals, the birthweight distributions were mismatched. In one institution, the proportion of infants weighing less than 1.5 kilograms at birth was 13 per cent of the total, while in another it was reported to be 100 per cent. Since the risk of developing RLF is inversely

Proportion of very small babies in RLF surveys of various hospitals

City	Years	No. of infants	RLF (per cent)	Birthweight under 1.5 kilograms (per cent)
		By cities and time periods (1922–48)		
Boston	1938–48	150	7	29
,,	1943–7	200	22	19
Providence	1941–7	225	7	13
Baltimore	1935–44	86	0	27
,,	1945–7	72	7	46
Hartford	1948	35	23	20
New York	1939–46	207	3	31
Cincinnati	1943–7	96	7	23
Birmingham	1945	104	0	20
Denver	1948	14	14	71
Chicago	1922–47	211	2	100

(Taken from the data assembled by Kinsey and Zacharias)

RLF in two hospitals (hypothetical)

	RLF in overall population at risk	RLF in two subgroups of overall population at risk	
	Birthweight < 2kg	Birthweight < 1.5kg	Birthweight 1.5-2kg
Hospital A	100 babies at risk / 8 / 8%	20 babies at risk / 4 / 20%	80 babies at risk / 4 / 5%
Hospital B	100 babies at risk / 17 / 17%	80 babies at risk / 16 / 20%	20 babies at risk / 1 / 5%

In Hospital A, RLF occurs in 8 per cent of 100 infants (birthweight under 2 kilograms); and the eye problem occurs in 17 per cent of 100 infants who are reared in Hospital B. The difference in distributions of birthweights within the under 2 kilograms class in these two hospitals accounts for the twofold *overall* difference in per cent occurrence of RLF; the rates within subgroup are identical in the two hospitals (under 1.5 kilograms = 20 per cent, 1.5–2 kilograms = 5 per cent).

related to the degree of prematurity as crudely judged by birthweight, relatively small differences in the distribution of birthweight would be expected to exert a magnified effect on the overall occurrence of RLF. When the experience in each hospital was examined in subgroups (by birthweight), some of the variation was reduced; but there was still considerable uncertainty about distortions related to other inequalities of babies in the various institutions.

Later surveys reporting associations between oxygen use and RLF were not consistent. Again, there was a strong suspicion that much of the inconsistency was related to differences in the compositions of the at-risk populations.

Circular definition of target population   Under the bewildering selective distributions of patients that exist in clinical medicine, the most conservative way to define the target population is to describe the *actual* collection of patients enrolled in a study. In effect we say, by a circular definition, that the results of the study are meant to apply to patients like those encountered in the study. And we proceed to describe the characteristics of 'patients enrolled' in some detail. A full description allows others to see the limits of the experience and the need for more information (for instance, how patients became available and how they were enrolled) before overstepping the narrow bounds of the reported experience.

Wide population base   Collaborative studies, involving a variety of institutions in one linked effort, are used to reduce the problems of uneven distribution of patients by providing a broad-based source of recruits. This potential was exploited in 1946 (p 44) when the pioneering tuberculosis treatment trial was conducted in Britain; patients enrolled in the trial were chosen from a parent population in eight tuberculosis hospitals throughout the country. A multicenter strategy was also attempted in order to deal with the hospital-to-hospital inconsistencies concerning oxygen treatment and RLF. In the national controlled clinical trial of 1953-4, 18 American hospitals treated small premature infants according to a prescribed experimental protocol; liberal oxygen use was compared with restricted oxygen treatment. The results of this study, one of the earliest large-scale controlled trials carried out in the United States, supported the positive association between generous use of oxygen and an increased risk of RLF. Doubts quickly faded away and the use of oxygen in the management of *all* premature infants throughout the world was sharply curtailed.

Unrepresentative patients in a controlled trial   I want to emphasize, since the point is often misunderstood, that random order of assignment in a treatment comparison trial does not solve the problem of *external* relevance.

The precaution improves the chances of internal representativeness (equal representation of participants in each of the treatment groups), but it does not increase the likelihood of drawing a representative sample of participants from the target population who are to be the beneficiaries of information acquired in the trial.

A striking example of the subtle ways in which systematic clustering of patients can occur was seen in the experience with a controlled study of the effectiveness of a treatment which was purported to reduce complications of pregnancy. Women enrolled in this trial were thought to represent a fair

Increased cancer risk among all participants in a controlled clinical trial

	Breast cancer (no.)	Occurrence[a] (per cent)	Risk ratio[b]
Exposed to DES	(32/693)	4.9	1.79
Unexposed to DES	(21/668)	3.1	
U.S. population[c]			1.00

[a] Participants in a double-blind study of the effectiveness of DES (diethylstilbestrol) in reducing the hazards of late complications of pregnancy (e.g. miscarriage), conducted in 1951–2. A total of 2162 enrolled in the study; 840 in the DES group and 806 in the non-medicated group completed the course of 'treatment'. During 1976–7, 693 mothers exposed and 668 not exposed to DES were interviewed by Bibbo and associates.
[b] Standardized incidence ratio adjusted for age distributions of women 'at risk' for breast cancer.
[c] The risk level of 1.00 was used as the base line for the general population as represented by the Connecticut Cancer Registry (incidence rates for the State of Connecticut—1963–5—are in good agreement with several United States and Canada data sources).

(Taken from the data of Bibbo and co-workers)

cross section of the at-risk pregnant population in the early 1950s. Years later it was found that the *daughters* of the women who received the treatment used in this trial (diethylstilbestrol, abbreviated DES) were developing cancer of the vagina at an alarming rate. As a result, the mothers who participated in the formal trial were contacted: Marluce Bibbo and coworkers at the University of Chicago found that those who had received DES treatment 25 years earlier experienced a relatively high rate of breast cancer. But this rate was only slightly higher than among concurrent controls who had been given no medication.

As it turned out, the entire group of women who were enrolled in this controlled trial had unrecognized (and inexplicable) similar characteristics which became manifest over the next quarter of a century: in the interim they developed breast cancer at a rate which was 1.79 times higher than the general population!

REPRESENTATION IN FOCUSED TRIALS

The uncertainties about representativeness can be narrowed if the scope of studies is scaled down to what John W. Tukey of Princeton University has called a 'focused clinical trial'. (This type of study is in contrast to a 'clinical inquiry' in which an intervention is postulated to help some class of patients, not specified in advance. From the collection of a great deal of information, the results are analyzed for each of many classes of patients— by age, sex, previous medical history, presenting symptoms, and prognosis, for example.) In the focused trial the class of patients to be considered is clearly specified *in advance*, Although the primary emphasis of the focused approach may remain pragmatic, a stated limit is placed on the practical goal.

Infants studied in the cooperative study of RLF

The 1953–4 national study of RLF, for example, was confined to the category of premature infants whose risk of blindness was most likely to be affected by a change in oxygen treatment policy: birthweight under 1.5 kilograms, age 2 days on enrollment (it was reasoned that early deaths would provide no information concerning the effect of treatment practices on RLF which develops many days and weeks after birth).

Source of patients As I have noted, this trial was conducted in 18 hospitals to achieve the goal of wide representation, but as we look more closely at the details, there were some sampling problems that are now evident with the clear vision of hindsight. Although the hospitals were located in different parts of the country, there was little variety in the type of institution; 16 of the 18 were university hospitals. The population of pregnant women in these referral centers was relatively atypical (many women with pregnancy complications were referred for specialized care and delivery). Additionally, many prematurely born infants were transferred to the large centers for expert attention (fully half of the more than 700 infants in the trial were in this category). All of the eligible babies in the participating hospitals were enrolled, but there was no assurance that these individuals, who were selected systematically before and after delivery, were 'typical' representatives of their class. What was needed, we see in retrospect, was a description of the characteristics of small, two-day-old premature infants who were *not* available to allow a comparison with participants.

Distribution of 'marker' characteristics All descriptions of patients' characteristics are only more or less complete, because we can never be sure that we know all, or even the most relevant, prognostic factors to judge 'representativeness.' Nonetheless, there is an indirect approach to the problem that provides some useful insights. We count the frequencies of a few easily identified 'markers' (for instance, gender, ethnicity, and the like) and examine their distribution in the class of patients under consideration.

In the national study, for example, we may approach the question of representativeness by examining the records of all participants *plus* a sample from community hospitals not included in the trial. The proportion of

Distribution of a 'marker' characteristic in a focused trial: Example of a format

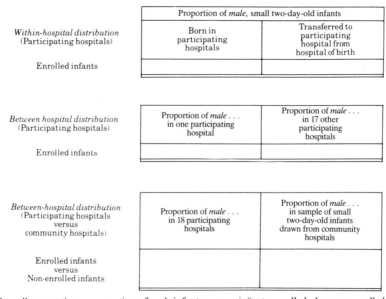

	Proportion of *male*, small two-day-old infants	
Within-hospital distribution (Participating hospitals)	Born in participating hospitals	Transferred to participating hospital from hospital of birth
Enrolled infants		

Between hospital distribution (Participating hospitals)	Proportion of *male* . . . in one participating hospital	Proportion of *male* . . . in 17 other participating hospitals
Enrolled infants		

Between-hospital distribution (Participating hospitals versus community hospitals)	Proportion of *male* . . . in 18 participating hospitals	Proportion of *male* . . . in sample of small two-day-old infants drawn from community hospitals
Enrolled infants versus Non-enrolled infants		

Overall proportion = proportion of *male* infants among infants enrolled plus non-enrolled sample from community hospitals

males, say, in the relatively wide-based population of at-risk babies provides an estimate of the proportion 'expected', and it may be compared with the proportions actually observed in each of the 18 participating hospitals. The distribution of the 'marker' provides a clue to the sorting of babies in the study; and we return for help with interpretation to the inanimate world of marbles and coins. The observed distribution of the proportion of male patients in each hospital may be compared with the frequency distribution pattern predicted by probability theory *if these groups were random samples* from the population of 'all' patients in the class. The differences between the proportions predicted and those observed may now be evaluated by reference to the laws of chance.

Vague warning of distortion

I should emphasize again that the arbitrarily chosen 'marker' characteristics may not be *the* important determinants with respect to outcome, but they serve as indicators of the amount of distortion that has occurred in the selection of patients. And unusual variations serve to warn that important (but unrecognized) variables may also be distributed in a way which distorts the results.

The sceptical approach is very much like that of the gambler who inspects a set of dice and finds that one is red and the other is green. Although the disparity in color may not influence the behavior of the dice, a high-roller is warned to withhold his bets until he has some assurance that he is playing with unbiased 'bones'.

ELIGIBILITY AND ENROLLMENT

All of the eligible infants admitted to participating hospitals were enrolled in the 1953-4 RLF trial, but that situation was atypical. Usually only a fraction of eligible candidates, those who agree voluntarily to participate or who are volunteered by surrogates, are actually enrolled. Needless to say, this process of selection by personal decision (influenced by family, friends, physicians, or by wordless fear) further complicates the murky issue of 'typical' representatives in medical studies.

There is simply no satisfactory way to resolve all of the uncertainties introduced when studies are conducted in patients who are selected on the basis of subjective criteria. Each extrapolation of results (from 'patients enrolled', to 'patients eligible', to 'patients in this class') is hemmed in with difficulties. Nevertheless, it is important to recognize the problems and to make some attempt to describe their scope. A full accounting of eligible patients who were *not* enrolled should be provided in reports of clinical studies with a warning that such missing patients may differ in some systematic way from participants. When there are many exclusions prior to enrollment in a clinical trial, generalization of results is seriously weakened by uncertainty.

Following all of the difficulties and limitations I have described in the recruitment and enrollment of representative participants in human studies, yet another block must be overcome—random order of allotments in a treatment comparison trial. It is this move which plays the most important role in assuring that like will be compared with like. The ramification of this controversy-ridden step in a controlled clinical trial will be discussed in the next chapter.

4 Controlled comparison

'HISTORICAL CONTROLS'

Most established treatments in the medical armamentarium were introduced without undergoing a formal test by concurrent comparison. The traditional approach has been to use the experience of the past as the basis for judging the effects of an innovation; 'historical controls' have served as the standards for comparisons. In recent times, physicians are becoming aware of the problems associated with retrospection, for it assumes that all important determinants except the new treatment under study have remained unchanged. Moreover, it assumes that all important determinants affecting outcome are known, so that the validity of the 'everything is the same' premise may be verified. The magnitude and complexity of these problems have grown as the pace of change in the modern world has quickened. Marvin A. Schneiderman of the National Cancer Institute, in the title of a review of the pitfalls in interpreting retrospective experience, asked (in exasperation), 'Looking backward: is it worth the crick in the neck?'

> 'And all our yesterdays have
> lighted fools the way to dusty death.'
> Shakespeare (*Macbeth*)

Changing course of illness

Major alterations in the 'natural' course of an illness may come about because of temporal changes in a variety of influences acting singly or in combination. These may include progressive alteration in social circumstances, the general health and nutritional status of patients, the degree of exposure to or inherent change in a pathologic agent, the criteria for diagnosis of the disease, the severity of the disorder, and the non-specific supportive care of patients, to name a few of the many variables that may change the course and final outcome of disease.

Trend of scarlet fever mortality

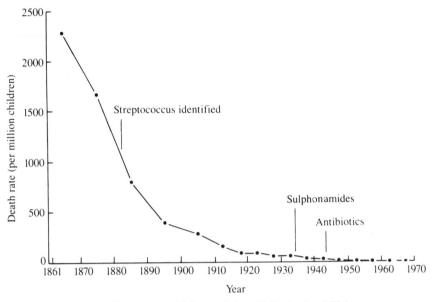

Death rates from scarlet fever among children under age 15, England and Wales
(Redrawn from McKeown's figure.)

Trend of mortality in scarlet fever The rapid decline in deaths caused by
one form of streptococcal infection, scarlet fever, is a striking example of
the problem in interpreting the effect of a medical innovation at a particular
moment in history. Thomas McKeown, the British epidemiologist, has
shown that approximately 90 per cent of the fall in the scarlet fever death
rate among children took place before the first use of what came to be
known as the 'miracle drugs' in 1935. And it is difficult to be sure whether
or not the rate of change since then has been influenced by modern antibacterial treatment.

Trend of mortality in tuberculosis Pulmonary tuberculosis in England and
Wales fell steadily in the 19th and the first half of the 20th century,
McKeown found. During this period many forms of treatment were used
with apparent success, but the claims are now considered to have been
exaggerated (treatment with gold salts, for example, was found to be worth-
less after it had been prescribed widely 'with good results' for over 15
years).

When the antibiotic agent, streptomycin, became available in 1946, members of the Medical Research Council in Britain were wary of scattered
reports indicating that the new treatment was effective against the ancient

Trend of pulmonary tuberculosis mortality

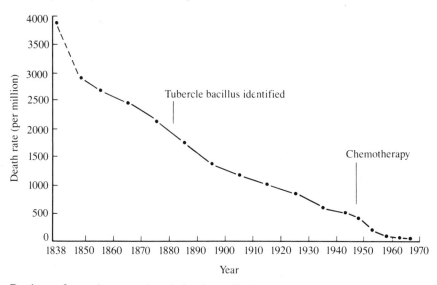

Death rates from pulmonary tuberculosis, all ages, England and Wales.
(Redrawn from McKeown's figure)

disease. They knew that the 'natural' course of the respiratory form of
tuberculosis was so variable and unpredictable it would be difficult to evaluate any mode of treatment. (The situation was in marked contrast to the
one in which the infection involved the central nervous system; meningeal
tuberculosis was uniformly fatal. Here the past was a reliable standard of
comparison. It was merely necessary to treat a group of proven cases; if
any recoveries took place this would be clear evidence that the new treatment was responsible for the unprecedented success.)

The multicenter randomized controlled trial organized in 1946 (p 37) set
out to compare results of the standard treatment for pulmonary tuberculosis (bed rest) with the experimental regimen (bed rest and streptomycin).
At the completion of the study it was found that mortality was lower
among patients who received the new drug. The need for a concurrent
control group in this landmark trial was underlined by the finding that
impressive clinical improvement occurred in some of the patients treated by
bed rest alone. Moreover, the limitations of streptomycin treatment also
became apparent. The new drug was toxic to the auditory nerve, and tub-
ercle bacilli quickly developed resistance to its antibacterial action.
Although the trial results suggested that the new treatment would accelerate
the decline in mortality rate from the respiratory form of tuberculosis, it was
also clear that a search for more satisfactory agents was urgently needed.

Demographic changes

Distortions in experiences may be introduced, as we have seen, by changes in the way patients are distributed throughout the medical system. Selective forces acting systematically, over time, on populations as a whole (such as changes in patterns of fertility) may also produce elusive changes in the types of patients available. Under these circumstances, it is difficult to evaluate the relative contribution of medical efforts, compared with in-tandem effects of social and demographic changes.

Shifts in high-risk births For example, beginning in the 1960s, there was a systematic shift in the distribution of births in the United States. The proportion of births among women in high-risk categories (that is, those with characteristics associated with high mortality in the offspring) began to decrease, and women with favorable outcome indicators accounted for a larger share of total births. A survey by Naomi M. Morris and her colleagues at the University of North Carolina noted the decline in infant mortality for the years 1965-72 and estimated that 27 per cent of the fall could be accounted for solely by the shifting proportions of characteristics in the pregnant population. The change was ascribed to 'family planning' (not family planning *services* necessarily, but individual decisions and be-havior concerning age at first pregnancy and number of pregnancies).

During the same years, projects were established in a number of Ameri-can cities to provide special prenatal and infant care. The success of these intensive efforts was measured by a fall in infant mortality rate. But, as the analysts pointed out, some of the improvement was related to more favor-able distributions of the inherent characteristics of childbearing women. Even under the most generous assumptions, only a small fraction of the decline in infant mortality seen in the country as a whole could possibly be attributed to the effectiveness of the well intentioned efforts to provide coordinated special care to a relatively small number of mothers and in-fants.

Conflicting effects of interventions

A major problem facing physicians is that of untangling multiple and, at times, opposing effects of their interventions. Unexpected harmful conse-quences of untried treatments are an ever present danger, and these may be difficult to detect when there is no concurrent control group of patients who receive the standard treatment.

Antibacterial treatment to prevent infection When antibacterial drugs be-came available after World War II, they were used with some encouraging results in newborn infants, but the record was disappointing in babies born prematurely who were at highest risk. The spotty results were thought to be related to the fact that early signs of bacterial invasion were difficult to recognize in the small babies.

Beginning in the late 1940s, premature infants were given antibacterial drugs to *prevent* infections, and survival seemed to improve following the introduction of this form of routine care. Almost five years elapsed before it was found, by means of a randomized controlled trial, that the new practice was not always benign. One established treatment regimen, penicillin plus sulfisoxazole, was found to have its intended effect of preventing fatal infections—but the beneficial action was irrelevant. In the formal trial, mortality rate after the second day of treatment was much higher among infants who received this established regimen that had been used widely with complete confidence. A non-infectious, often fatal, form of brain damage (known as kernicterus) was found nine times more often among babies who succumbed after the accepted treatment than among concurrent controls treated with a newly proposed drug to stave off infection.

The fatal side effect of the established treatment was unsuspected and had been completely overlooked before the formal trial. An increase in kernicterus-related deaths during the years of penicillin/sulfisoxazole treatment was hidden among other fatal conditions (often multiple in the same baby) found commonly at the time of autopsy examination. (It was later discovered by Gerald B. Odell, then at Johns Hopkins University, that sulfisoxazole 'released' the protein-bound yellow pigment, bilirubin, in the blood of jaundiced newborns; the toxic pigment was then free to enter and fatally damage the brain of a treated baby.)

A biblical comparative trial involving children

The prophet Daniel conducted a trial of a vegetarian diet (a pottage of leguminous plants and water) as compared with a daily provision of the king's meat which was offered to a group of well-favored children 'such as had ability in them to stand in the king's palace.' At the end of ten days on the experimental diet, 'their countenances appeared fairer and fatter in flesh than all the children which did eat the portion of the king's meat.'

Daniel 1:11–15

RANDOMIZED ALLOTMENT

The sulfisoxazole incident is not unique. It is a tragic reminder of what is, in fact, the rightful burden of all innovation: How can the risk of introducing a new treatment be limited? Despite the most extensive pre-clinical study, the first human application of a powerful treatment is a blind gamble. The possibilities of gain and loss must be undertaken without fore-knowledge of the probable odds. How is the 'impossible' decision made to choose between the accepted standard treatment and the proposed improved approach when a fellow human being must be assigned to one of the two (or more) treatments under test?

John Wesley draws lots to seek guidance concerning marriage (March 4, 1737)

'Having both of us [Mr Delamotte and himself] sought God by deep consideration, fasting and prayer, in the afternoon we conferred together but could not come to any decision. We both apprehended Mr Ingham's objection to be the strongest, the doubt whether she was what she appeared. But this doubt was too hard for us to solve. At length we agreed to appeal to the Searcher of Hearts. I accordingly made three lots. In one was writ, "Marry": in the second "Think not of it this year". After we had prayed to God to "give a perfect lot", Mr Delamotte drew the third, in which were the words, "Think of it no more". Instead of the agony I had reason to expect I was enabled to say cheerfully "Thy will be done". We cast lots again to know whether I ought to converse with her any more, and the direction I received from God was "Only in the presence of Mr Delamotte".'

(Quoted from Wesley's journal by F.N. David of the University of London)

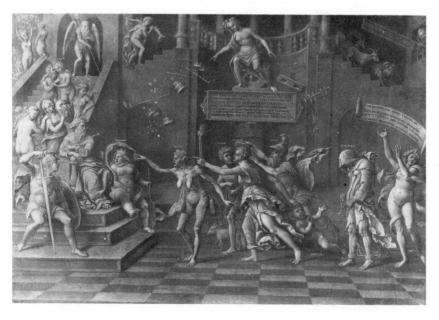

Allegory of Fortune
Fortune is often portrayed on a ball or a wheel, often with a blindfold. The wheel is usually introduced in pictures as a symbol of uncertainty or insecurity. In this painting by Leombruno (16th century), the goddess is characterized as inconstant, dangerous, and delicately balanced (*Dea varia, lubrica et fragilis*).

Limiting risk by lot

A solution is to be found by turning to one of the most venerable practices in the long history of humankind: in the face of an irresolvable dilemma the gods are consulted for guidance. Sortilege, or divination by lots, is the time-honored and eminently fair method used to guide choices under conditions in which there is paralyzing uncertainty. Many variations in detail have been used, but the general procedure is fairly uniform; the question is posed, the lot is cast, and the decision is made. The method, it has been noted, does not give the god, or more specifically the goddess of fortune, much scope for self-expression, but at least it produces an unequivocal directive. And in medicine, I must add, the method protects patients from the consequences of the all too human frailties of their caretakers.

Randomization

The ancient method of divination by lot is formalized in the present-day method of randomization of treatments. The procedure was invented (p 11) to ensure that compared treatments will be assigned to patients in such a way that all possible allocations are equally likely within the constraints of the experimental design. (One such restriction is used in a method called 'balanced' randomization in which the numbers of assignments are equalized in small blocks of consecutive patients.)

Advantages of random allotment   The essential weakness of before-and-after design is overcome in a randomized clinical trial. Both standard treatment and new treatment groups are observed concurrently, thus eliminating the 'time bias' of historic controls. And random allotment eliminates the physician's bias in the assignment of treatments. It has been pointed out, for example, that biased assignment of patients is particularly likely to occur in selective comparisons of medical versus surgical treatments; often only low risk patients are considered to be candidates for operations whereas many more candidates are judged suitable for medical treatments.

The precaution of random allotment ensures that neither personal idiosyncrasies nor lack of balanced judgment enters into the formation of different treatment groups. It removes the unfairness that may arise when treatments are prescribed on the basis of unjustified guesses. Of course, the protective plan may be foiled if patients are enrolled only on condition that they receive a specified treatment (or if they are removed when the goddess of fortune decides against one of the prejudged alternatives). A decision to participate must be made before the treatment assignment is disclosed if a patient is to be shielded fairly when taking a risky step into the unknown.

Another advantage of random assignment is that the method tends to

'Balanced' randomization sequences

Balanced randomization should be considered when enrollment in a trial takes place slowly over a period of months or years because temporal changes in severity of illness are not uncommon. The object of the approach is to ensure fairly equal matching of numbers in treatment groups at all times in the course of a prolonged trial. For example, two treatments (A and B) may be assigned in a restricted form of randomization that enforces equal numbers at the enrollment of every sixth patient. All of the 20 possible sequences of 3A's and 3B's are given number designations as follows:

Number	Sequence	Number	Sequence
00–04	AAABBB	50–54	BAAABB
05–09	AABABB	55–59	BAABAB
10–14	AABBAB	60–64	BAABBA
15–19	AABBBA	65–69	BABAAB
20–24	ABAABB	70–74	BABABA
25–29	ABABAB	75–79	BABBAA
30–34	ABABBA	80–84	BBAAAB
35–39	ABBAAB	85–89	BBAABA
40–44	ABBABA	90–94	BBABAA
45–49	ABBBAA	95–99	BBBAAA

Number category 00–04 indicates that the compared treatments will be given to six consecutive patients in the order AAABBB, category 05–09 designates the order AA-BABB, and so on. A series of two-digit numbers are then obtained from a random number table and these determine the sequence of six treatment blocks in the trial. Each treatment assignment is placed in an opaque envelope and these are arranged in a long series according to the treatment order in consecutive blocks. The envelopes are sealed and the face of each envelope marked with a number to indicate the order in which the envelopes are to be opened as consecutive patients are enrolled and treated. When six patients are enrolled, the numerical balance between treatment A and treatment B is equal, and the equality is maintained with the enrollment of the twelfth, eighteenth … patient.

Since the assignment for the last person entered in each block can be determined before the envelope is opened, the ideal of 'masked' treatment decision is not met completely. The potential for such disclosure can be reduced by varying the size of consecutive sets. A random order of block size makes it very difficult to determine the next assignment in a series.

balance treatment groups in respect to relevant determinants of outcome, whether or not these factors are known. (Such blind faith is related to our convictions about the behavior of random processes: rain drops *do* tend to fall equally on exposed squares of paper). And, finally, randomization guarantees the validity of the statistical tests of 'significance' that are used to compare treatments.

The latter arguments deserve special emphasis because the need for the treatment-by-lot step in bedside studies is often misunderstood. For example, comparisons of treatments using concurrent controls often are thought to be impractical because it is virtually impossible to assemble two groups of patients that are matched exactly in every clinical detail. When R.A. Fisher introduced the element of randomization in experimental design, he explained that it is pointless to insist that all conditions in compared groups must be exactly alike because the list of possible factors that might influence the outcome can never be exhausted: *the number is unknown*. Random assignment of treatments serves as the fundamental safeguard under these conditions of uncertainty about risk variables. Although the groups compared are never perfectly matched for 'all important determinants,' the process of randomization fulfills the requirements of the logic of chance.

Laws of chance operate   On the assumption that the results are governed by the laws of chance, we may ascribe a probability distribution to the difference in outcome *expected* between groups receiving equally effective treatments. Any *observed* difference may now be described in the terms of 'betting odds' used by gamblers. As has been emphasized by David P. Byar of the National Cancer Institute, it is the process of randomization that generates the 'statistical significance' test (p 127), and this process is independent of prognostic factors known or unknown. The validity of 'significance' levels based on randomization does not require the unachievable assumption that the treatment groups are exactly matched.

Stratification and sensitivity   Contrived efforts to achieve near equality in compared groups are often made before randomization by subdividing eligible patients into subgroups of individuals who resemble each other in respect to their known prospects for illness outcome. The ideal sought by the tactic, called prognostic stratification, is to reduce the variability of outcomes and increase the sensitivity of a trial. It is less likely that a specific effect will be overlooked when comparisons are made between individuals under similar risk. For example, the gradient of birthweight-related risk of RLF was so steep that infants enrolled in the national study were divided into three risk strata (by birthweight) and random allotments of treatments were carried out among babies within each stratum.

Practical limits of subgroups   As a practical matter, the number of prognostic characteristics that can be considered is severely limited by the inherent diseconomy of scale in the problem. The addition of each extra variable means that the number of mutually exclusive subgroups will increase geometrically. For example, two variates require four subgroups, three require eight and so on. Many enrollees are needed if each of the subgroups is to have enough members to provide a reasonable contrast. As a result, the number of prognostic categories for assignments in clinical trials is usually scaled down to take into account only the most important determinants thought to have a bearing on the outcome of the study. Sometimes, a summary prognostic index based on several characteristics may be used as a single variable for assignments. This may achieve a reasonable balance among the separate factors on which the index was formulated.

There is some disagreement about the need for stratified entry in large single center trials; in the alternative approach, prognostic stratification is carried out only at the time of analysis of results. In multicenter trials, the characteristics of patients in each hospital are likely to vary in ways which may affect outcome. Thus, it is advisable to consider each center as a replication of the trial and to randomize accordingly; stratification by hospital is a minimum subdivision in collaborative studies.

Random allotment within prognostic strata

The randomized clinical trial of two oxygen-management regimens was conducted in 18 hospitals throughout the United States. All premature infants who weighed 1.5 kilograms or less and who survived 48 hours, born in or brought to the cooperating hospitals, were admitted to the study. A Coordination Center in Detroit, Michigan was notified by telegram of the enrollment of each infant and assignments were made as follows*:

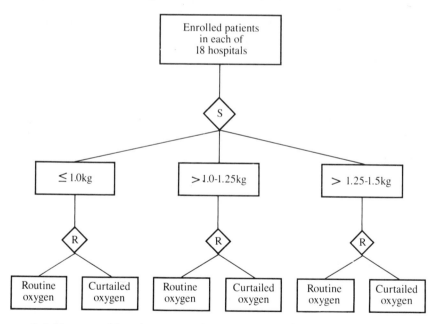

S: babies grouped into three prognostic strata according to birthweight (under 1.0 kilogram, 1.0 to 1.25 kilograms, and 1.25 to 1.5 kilograms)

R: random allocations to oxygen management regimens (routine oxygen treatment or curtailed oxygen administration)

At the end of the trial, outcomes in each of the oxygen management subgroups were added for a final comparison of results.

*Allocation in the trial was more involved than indicated here because of a two-stage design (p 177), but the principle of random allotment within subgroups was preserved.

A caveat   Having made the arguments for the importance of the 'casting of lots,' I must now pass along Feinstein's warning against undue reverence for randomization as a panacea for the cure or prevention of all intellectual maladies in planning clinical studies. Obviously, it would be misleading to imply that distortions do not occur with random allotments. The laws of chance require that gross imbalances, like all improbable events, must occur in the long run.

ALLOCATION IN PILOT TRIALS

Pilot observations of the results of a new treatment (to determine the dosage and other details of administration) are usually carried out in selected patients. Randomization starts only after these initial explorations have been completed in enough people to allow a formal trial to be carried out without changes in a prescribed regimen.

Randomize the first patient

The standard approach has been challenged by Thomas C. Chalmers, of the Mount Sinai School of Medicine, who has proposed that randomization should begin with the first patient. He argues that the limitation-of-risk rationale for random allotment can be defended when there is no hint about relative efficacy and toxicity of a new drug (or procedure): this innocent state exists in its purest form at the time the first patient is to be treated. What the clinical investigator is doing in an uncontrolled pilot trial, he continues, is asking certain patients to forego their right to the standard accepted therapy and be treated by a procedure that has not yet been developed sufficiently to warrant its comparison with that standard treatment. Chalmers' arguments are logical and quite practical: a stepwise approach, ending in a final version of the randomized trial, can be carried out with due regard for the rights of patients and the requirements of the rules of evidence. But it must be firmly resolved that the investigative efforts will not end with pilot observations.

Uncontrolled pilot studies

Preliminary results of success or of failure are frequently misleading when initial observations are conducted without concurrent controls. If the pilot experience fails to demonstrate the hoped-for effect, efforts are often abandoned before a potentially useful intervention is given a fair trial and the preliminary results are rarely reported. On the other hand, if the initial results indicate a positive effect, the results are published and the investigators become so convinced of the value of the intervention that they are unwilling to conduct a critical trial to determine the limits of applicability of the new treatment.

It has become customary in preliminary reports to include a paragraph advising that controlled studies should be carried out to confirm the initial observations. Such trials, however, are rarely, if ever, conducted by the original, enthusiastic innovator. The report of encouraging results has a ripple effect; others are emboldened to conduct uncontrolled explorations of the hopeful approach and a critical test is delayed.

The history of a surgical procedure to prevent bleeding from varicosities of the esophagus complicating cirrhosis of the liver is an example of a frequently seen relationship between the design of studies and expressed enthusiasm for new treatments. After 15 years of controversy concerning the treatment to prevent esophageal hemorrhage, a large-scale randomized clinical trial was conducted by a cooperative group of Boston hospitals. No

Design of studies and expressed enthusiasm

'... nothing improves the performance of an innovation as much as the lack of controls.'
Hugo Muench

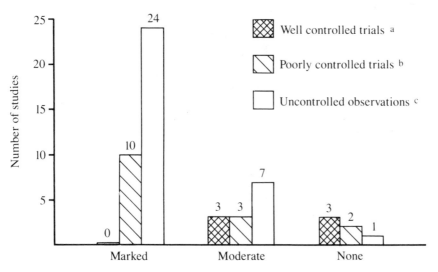

Degree of enthusiasm for treatment*

*Enthusiasm for a surgical treatment purported to reduce the risk of esophageal hemorrhage in cirrhosis of the liver (53 studies of the procedure reviewed by John P. Gilbert and his associates at Harvard University).

[a] Well controlled: a study in which assignment to treatment groups is in random order and the patient is accepted for study before the treatment is known.

[b] Poorly controlled: a study in which there is selection of patients for the treatments to be compared according to clinical judgment, and comparison is made with the whole group or the unselected group; or a study in which the controls are historical and originate in a different time or place.

[c] Uncontrolled: no attempt is made to compare the patients receiving the treatment in question with a group not receiving this treatment.

evidence of a beneficial effect of the surgical procedure could be detected. I will return to the issues raised by pilot observations in Chapter 9 (The Stopping Rule).

Two definitions

Quasi-Experimental Design
The phrase 'quasi-experimental design,' according to D.L. Sills in the *International Encyclopedia of the Social Sciences*, refers to the application of an experimental mode of analysis and interpretation to bodies of data not meeting the full requirements of experimental control. The circumstances in which it is appropriate are those of experimentation in social settings—including planned interventions—where complete experimental control is not possible. When properly done, when attention is given to the specific implications of the weaknesses of the design in question, quasi-experimental analysis can provide a valuable extension of the experimental method.

True Experimentation
The core requirement of a true experiment lies in the experimenter's ability to apply experimental treatments in complete independence of the prior states of the persons under study. This independence makes the resulting differences interpretable as effects of the differences in treatment. The independence of experimental treatment from prior status is assured by randomization in assignments to treatments. Where innovations are to be introduced throughout a social system and where the introduction cannot in any event be simultaneous, a use of randomization in the staging can provide an experimental comparison of the new and the old, using groups receiving the delayed introduction as controls.

NON-RANDOM ASSIGNMENT

The term 'quasi-experimental' has been used to describe non-random methods for assigning compared treatments. In the simplest of these, standard treatment and new treatment are assigned alternately as patients appear for enrollment. This systematic method (and variations, such as assignment by alternate day, by odd or even hospital chart number, and so on) offers no protection against the introduction of personal biases that might interfere with the basic goal of comparing like with like. For example, physicians may deliberately 'steer' patients into a preferred group when they know the schedule of assignments. Moreover, even when they conscientiously try to avoid influencing assignments, they may unwittingly do so when they decide whether or not their patients are qualified for enrollment in the trial. If these decisions are made when they know which treatment the patients are to receive, it is difficult to avoid selective recruitment. The result is a systematic sorting of patients that may have a much greater influence on outcome than the treatments under test.

ADAPTIVE ALLOCATION PROCEDURES

A number of assignment schemes have been developed that use information obtained during the course of a clinical trial to determine the treatment prescribed for the next patient who is enrolled. Some of the approaches seek progressive improvement in the balance of numbers and prognostic characteristics, others adjust allocations according to the responses to previously assigned treatments in the hope of winning in what might be considered a game against nature.

Marvin Zelen of Harvard described a game-like design that uses the 'play the winner rule', well known in gambling. A success of one treatment in a comparative series generates a future trial of the same treatment with a new patient; a failure generates a future trial of the alternative treatment. In practice, the first treatment is assigned by the toss of a coin. If the response is successful the 'winning' treatment is offered to successive patients until a failure occurs. At that point the alternative treatment is used for the next candidate. When a failure is encountered on the alternative, the next patient receives the original 'winner' and so on.

Another adaptive plan, known as the 'two armed bandit' method, begins by assigning treatments in random order. As the trial proceeds, information is gained about the probability of success for each treatment. The new data is used to adjust the ratios of assignments, so that a progressively higher proportion of newly enrolled patients receives the currently 'better' treatment.

Shortcomings of adaptive designs

The general aims of adaptive strategies for treatment assignments cannot be faulted. They are used to increase the chance that more patients will be assigned to the superior treatment as the trial progresses and to shorten a trial in which some patients are exposed to an inferior treatment. Unfortunately, there are a number of practical difficulties that limit the usefulness of the approach. In chronic disorders, for example, there may be a long delay (years) between treatment and outcome. Moreover, the response used to judge the 'winning' treatment may be misleading if unexpected serious complications turn up later (for instance, liberal oxygen treatment was found to improve the respiratory performance of premature infants while long afterward the link between the intervention and RLF was uncovered). Finally, a serious limitation of adaptive schemes arises from the shaky assumption that patients admitted throughout the study are homogeneous in characteristics which affect the outcome of treatment.

Dilemmas of allocating untried treatments

Undoubtedly, there will be continued efforts to seek improvements in the designs for allocating treatments in clinical trials. And there is no reason to expect that a single approach will be suitable for all clinical studies. It is unrealistic to ignore the fact that some doctors and their patients are unwilling to submit treatment decisions to the luck of the draw. Nevertheless, the random assignment format remains the most powerful one available for comparisons of treatments. And, I wish to re-emphasize, the dilemmas for each individual patient enrolled in a randomized trial and for the community as a whole are resolved by one of the fairest risk-limiting practices used by human societies. The democratic aspect of this approach to containment of hazards was demonstrated in the randomized clinical trial of sulfisoxazole treatment of babies. It was shocking to find the fatal complication in those who were enrolled in the trial, but the new information was obtained by a strategy that spared half of the participants from exposure to the unsuspected hazard of the previously 'accepted' treatment and would spare the lives of future babies.

The modern version of sortilege affirms an ancient observation: Man has one thing in view, Fate has another.

> 'Cry and howl, son of man ...
> Because *it is* a trial ...
> Thou therefore, son of man, prophecy, and smite
> thine hands together ...
> Go thee one way or other ... withersoever thy *face* is set.
> I will also smite mine hands together and I will cause
> my fury to rest: I the LORD have said *it*.'
>
> *Ezekiel* 21:12–17

5 Intervention

A tribal medicine man never teaches an apprentice quite the whole of his knowledge. Allopathic healers, on the other hand, are slowly shedding the cloak of mystery as they go about the business of intervening in the 'natural' course of the ills that befall us. Understandably, there is wistful reluctance on the part of physicians (and their patients) to reduce the therapeutic act to a visible formula. But dispassionate evaluation cannot begin until medical maneuvers are described fully.

SPECIFIED MANEUVERS

In a formal clinical trial, both the standard treatment and the innovation must be specified. The alternatives need to be stated in sufficient detail to permit others to repeat the maneuvers with precision, for it is the everyday application of the results of bedside studies that must be kept in view.

The standard regimen

The 'established' treatment is often difficult to pin down. Most regimens have been introduced informally, and variations on a therapeutic theme are the rule rather than the exception. Nonetheless, a consensus needs to be obtained about the orthodox approach for two reasons. First, if the trial is to be perceived as a proper challenge to accepted treatment, there should be few doubts that this standard was fairly represented. Second, if the sought-for contrast between treatments is to be made as sharp as possible, there should be an effort to reduce the irregularity of results. A compromise should be effected between the need to conduct a trial that is not far removed from everyday practice of medicine and the need to reduce the blurring effects of a loosely defined standard of treatment.

Oxygen monitoring in the RLF trial The 'standard oxygen treatment' of premature infants in the national study of RLF, for example, was defined as supplemental oxygen administered in a concentration over 50 per cent from age 2 days to age 30 days. This stipulation formalized the custom of routine oxygen administration that had been used widely for years prior to the study in the management of small infants. However, the specified version of the convention called for measurement of the concentration of oxygen in incubators at eight-hour intervals. Since the clinical instruments for measuring this concentration easily and reliably had become available only a short time before the study began, the 'standard practice' as carried out in the study was not the usual practice followed in hospitals throughout the Western world; it was a regulated representation of the accepted approach.

The loss of realism and the gain in precision sharpened the comparison with the new proposal ('curtailed oxygen'—stipulated as use of the supplemental gas only as needed to relieve symptoms of oxygen lack, concentration not to exceed 50 per cent). But artificiality of the 'tight' plan exacted a price: extrapolation of the results of the study had to be made with considerable caution, particularly since the difference in treatment detail between study and everyday practice was not academic. It was later found that prolonged exposure to non-fluctuating concentrations of oxygen was needed to produce abnormal changes in the retinal blood vessels of experimental animals.

Uniform technical performance   When interventions involve technical skills, the problem of developing a uniform standard is particularly difficult. The

Wide range of outcomes in cancer surgery

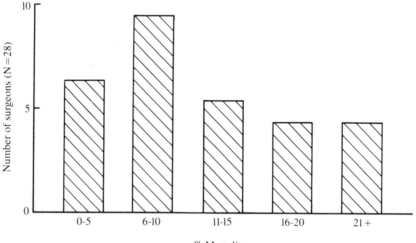

% Mortality

Mortality among 932 patients with cancer of the large bowel in a multicenter trial of surgical excision; the data were collected by L.P. Fielding and other surgeons at St Mary's Hospital Medical School (London). The wide range of post-operative mortality reported by 28 surgeons (each of whom contributed 10 or more patients) suggests that outcomes were to a considerable degree surgeon-dependent.

'same' surgical operation may have widely different outcomes in the hands of different surgeons. Similar problems arise when the non-specific effects of the 'healer' influence outcome (p 66).

It should be recognized, however, that the vagaries here are not unique in any qualitative sense. To a greater or lesser degree, the limitations imposed by irregularities in the therapeutic maneuver are a part of all clinical studies. Although the conflict between the demands of realism and those of order can never be completely resolved, it is important to take the time to develop a plan that will narrow the gap.

Bona fide treatments

Many clinical trials yield 'negative' results; the difference in outcome between groups receiving the standard treatment and others who are treated with the innovation is no greater than would be expected to occur frequently by chance. It is a challenge to planners to increase the amount of information that can be gleaned from a negative result, for there is a strong obligation to patient participants to ensure that a treatment trial is, quite literally, bona fide. The treatments compared should be alternatives that are offered *in good faith* that the results will be relevant to the welfare of those enrolled. Moreover, the predicted outcomes should have substantial implications that bear on current theoretical and applied problems.

Richard Peto of Oxford University has suggested several questions to be posed when planning treatment trials. What value will the results have if both treatment groups fare equally well? Can the design be altered to make a negative result even more valuable? A drug trial, for example, is always a test of the drug in the particular dose and manner given, not a trial of the drug *per se*. Distinctive comparisons, such as determining the largest dose of a new agent that can be given safely, provide more meaningful negative results than less marked contrasts.

Treatment of incipient RLF An instructive 'negative' experience took place in 1950 when the newly available drug ACTH (adrenocorticotropic hormone, which produces heightened activity of the adrenal gland) was used in a desperate attempt to halt the early blood vessel changes of RLF. Following very encouraging results in a pilot experience involving 31 infants, the potent agent was evaluated in a randomized clinical trial.

The formal test results indicated that the new treatment was completely ineffective in preventing blindness, and it appeared quite unlikely that this failure to confirm the preliminary findings could be explained by inadequate dosage of ACTH. All of the treated infants experienced temporary retardation of body growth, and the occurrence of serious infections (a feared complication of prolonged adrenal gland stimulation) was higher than in untreated controls.

This disheartening 'negative' trial revealed that early changes of RLF usually subside spontaneously (a previously unsuspected finding that was supported by observations reported two years later). Additionally, the trial had the immediate positive effect of protecting half of the enrolled infants from the risk of exposure to the potent hormone. And the discouraging experience served to warn others about the dangers of this fruitless approach to the prevention of blindness.

Dosage of treatment agents

The problems of flexible dosage in treatment trials are not easily solved: particularly when the end point for potency is difficult to define, when there are technical difficulties in monitoring on going effects, and when there are multiple effects that must be taken into account. In the national RLF trial many of these difficulties were recognized—in retrospect.

Oxygen dosage in the RLF trial   It was decided in the oxygen-and-RLF trial that 50 per cent oxygen concentration in inspired air would serve as the boundary between the two management regimens. This ceiling was chosen for the 'curtailed oxygen treatment' group because it was believed (in the early 1950s) that concentrations in the range of 40–50 per cent were adequate for relief in infants who required treatment with this life-supporting gas. The higher concentrations specified for 'standard' management acknowledged the established practice of keeping very small infants in highly enriched environments on the assumption that this regimen improved respiratory performance, thereby reducing the risk of death and of brain damage in survivors.

Oxygen concentration on either side of the 50 per cent demarcation line was not specified by protocol; in fact, a wide range of concentrations was used. The duration of treatment in the 'curtailed-use' group was on an 'as needed' basis (length of exposure varied from zero to as long as three weeks). When the results of the trial indicated that the risk of RLF was reduced with no apparent increase in mortality among infants who received curtailed amounts of oxygen, many questions surfaced about the relationship between dosage and outcome. For example: Does the risk of RLF increase with rising concentrations of oxygen, with longer durations of exposure, or with some function of concentration and duration? Most important was the question: What is the risk of eye damage when oxygen is administered only during the first two days of life, the period excluded in the trial?

The large body of information collected in the study of more than 700 babies provided an opportunity for a 'data-dredging' search to formulate very specific hypotheses concerning the dosage of oxygen and outcome. And the sifting operation was, indeed, carried out; it was observed, for instance, that RLF occurred more frequently with increasing duration of exposure, but not with increasing concentration of oxygen. The weakness of such associations, however, was self-evident in the trial design: incremental differences in oxygen exposure (within the two broadly stated treatment prescriptions) were made not by lot but according to individual judgments of treating doctors. The connection between dosage and RLF risk was completely undermined by uncertainty about confounding influences; the sickest babies received oxygen treatment for the longest periods and in the highest concentrations within the wide limits defined in the trial protocol.

Urgently needed tests of the unsolved questions concerning oxygen dosage simply could not be undertaken in babies because of ethical constraints. And studies in other species did not resolve the problems. Although early changes of RLF could be produced, blindness did not occur in experimental animals exposed to oxygen.

In the years following the announcement, in 1954, of the RLF trial results, the questions concerning the exact relationships between oxygen dosage and the well being of premature infants became more complex.

Cerebral palsy and RLF

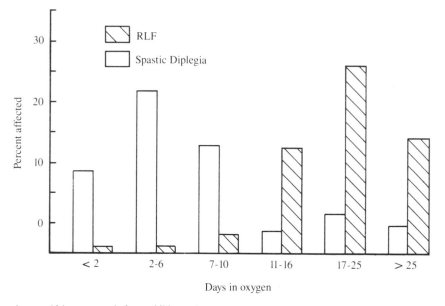

Among 194 prematurely-born children who received oxygen treatment, cerebral palsy (spastic diplegia) occurred more frequently with short than with long exposures. A reverse trend was noted for RLF.
(From the report of Alison D. McDonald)

Surveys of treatment practices suggested a conflict of outcomes with oxygen curtailment. Short exposures to supplemental oxygen were accompanied by relatively low frequencies of RLF, but spastic diplegia (a form of cerebral palsy) was found to occur more often with curtailed treatments. Additional doubts about the overly simple extrapolations concerning oxygen dosage were triggered by surveys of the trend of mortality among premature infants. The curtailed oxygen practice beginning in the mid-1950s was followed by a halt in the downward trend in mortality rates of babies under 1 day of age. The important question raised by these disturbing observations was: How do the *intertwined* risks of death, brain damage, and RLF blindness vary with increasing exposure to supplemental oxygen?

It was reasonable to postulate, for example, that at the cost of minimal increase in the risk of RLF, there would be a large reduction in the risk of brain damage and of death for infants exposed to doses of supplemental oxygen that lie between the extremes formally tested in the national trial. But ethical barriers, once more, made it impossible to test the thesis rigorously. The issues remain unresolved to the present day.

Limitations of a single trial

The prolonged uncertainties in the use of a familiar substance, oxygen, for an everyday problem such as the management of newborn babies, are not particularly unique. These kinds of complexities are commonplace in the evaluation of interventions in medicine. It is unreasonable to expect to settle all of the important questions concerning treatments with a single well planned trial. Initial decisions about new therapies almost always need to be modified, and it is realistic to plan, from the outset, that a *series* of trials will be required to bring the boundaries of efficacy and the magnitudes of trade-off risks into focus. The plodding pace of clinical trials is so frustrating that there is a strong temptation to wring as much meaning as possible from each experience in the hope of avoiding additional or phased formal tests. Unfortunately, as in the RLF experience, the short cuts are full of unexpected traps.

EVENHANDED TREATMENT

It is completely unrealistic to expect that clinical trials can be carried out by neutral investigators who are not 'betting' on the final results. Personal bias is a given in all studies and it is necessary to devise fairly elaborate schemes to thwart or, at least, diminish its effects.

'Masking'

The infelicitious term 'double blind' refers to the strategy in which neither the physician nor his patient knows which of the alternative treatments under test has been given. Although this guarantees that the treatments will be administered with an even hand and that observation of results will be unbiased, there are a number of practical difficulties that limit the approach. The disguise may be imperfect or, as in surgical treatment, it may be impossible to achieve. Additionally, it creates workaday problems (especially adjustment of dosage) that are difficult to overcome. And the artificial trial conditions are completely different from those of the real world to which the results are meant to apply.

Other safeguards to ensure objectivity in the application of treatments and in observation of results, such as using third party observers who do not know which treatment the patient received, have advantages over highly contrived measures that keep the physician from knowing which treatment has been prescribed. The term 'single blind' is used when one of the parties is kept from recognizing treatments and the 'masked' class (treating physician, observer, or patient) should be specified.

Experimenters' effects

Although it is not always possible to devise a practical 'masking' plan, the consequences of experimenter bias are not easily dismissed. Two major types of influence need to be considered; both are usually unintentional. The first operates 'in' the observer without modifying the response of patients (the effects, to be discussed in Chapter 6, are felt in the notation of phenomena). The second type of experimenter's effect is interactional. It modifies the actual response of patients to maneuvers and thus can be considered to be an element of these interventions.

The physician component of treatment   There is evidence (especially in behavioral research) that the experimenter's orientation leads to interaction with subjects in ways that increase the likelihood that the response will confirm the proposed hypothesis. In medical settings, physicians tend to offer patients cues about what is expected through voice quality and non-verbal body behavior, even though the content of instruction is standardized. The biasing effects of such cues on the responses of patients are not entirely controlled by shutting off communication, as nearly all people have learned ways of acting in the presence of authoritative figures. The self-fulfilling prophecy effects are exaggerated by psychosocial influences: experimenters high in status tend to obtain more conforming responses from their subjects than do lowly researchers.

The personality of the experimenter may influence the results of behavioral research: friendly examiners administering standardized tests of intelligence are likely to obtain better intellectual performance than are more aloof examiners or those who are perceived as threatening or strange by examinees. These phenomena have been summarized by the phrase 'the demand characteristics of the experimental situation' which include all of the cues which govern subjects' perceptions of their roles and the investigator's hypothesis.

When patients trust their physicians they act in ways that are meant to please; compliant patients have a remarkably intuitive ability to sense what is wanted of them and they provide it. In long-term studies, participants often come to identify with researchers and their aims and feel obliged to conform as a self-imposed condition for maintaining the bond. In follow-up studies of children, for example, mothers' caretaking behavior may be favorably influenced by researchers, and this becomes an unevaluated co-intervention that alters the outcome-of-interest in the child.

The expectancy phenomenon   The effects of investigator's expectations have been tested extensively by social psychologists, notably Robert Rosenthal

Effect of experimenter's expectancy on maze learning in rats

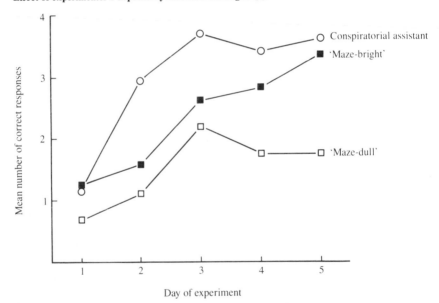

Day of experiment

In Rosenthal's investigation a group of students were given written instructions concerning an experiment in rats. They were told that continuous in-breeding had led to a strain which was considerably better than 'normal' rats in maze learning ability; these rats were labeled 'maze-bright;' another strain was 'maze-dull,' the students were told. The rats were, in fact, ordinary rats and they were assigned in random order to thirteen groups, five animals in each group. Six students conducted maze-learning 'runs' with 'maze-bright' rats, six used 'maze-dull' animals, and a research assistant who knew the truth conducted 'runs' on the thirteenth group of animals (she was instructed to get as good performance from her animals as possible without violating the formally programmed procedures). Each rat was 'run' for 10 trials per day over a 5 day period. When the animals turned into the darker of two platforms of a T-maze, they were rewarded and the response was scored 'correct.'

of Harvard University. He has found that experimenters may change during the course of their experiments under the influence of responses obtained from the first few enrollees. When the first few subjects react according to expectations, the behavior of experimenters is modified in ways which influence subsequent subjects to conform to the prediction of the hypothesis.

In one trial, the expectancy phenomenon was evaluated by 'creating' researchers who differed only in the expectations they held about the result of a specific experiment involving laboratory animals. The participants were given rats that were to be taught to run a maze with the aid of visual clues. Some were told that their rats had been specifically bred for 'maze brightness'; others were told that their rats were 'maze dull'; and a research assistant was told the truth: the groups of rats had been formed by random assignment from a common pool. The assistant was urged to obtain a good performance from her animals. At the end of a five-day trial, the results indicated that rats assigned to experimenters expecting brighter behavior showed better learning compared to rats given to investigators expecting dull performance. The conspiratorial assistant obtained the best results of all. The experience suggested that the experimenter who was urged to obtain good performance from animal subjects achieved even better performance than others who were biased to *expect* good performance but were not explicitly instructed to obtain it.

If rats became brighter when expected to by an investigator, it seemed possible that children might become more intelligent when expected to by their teacher. 'The Pygmalion Experiment' was conducted among elementary school children and the results supported the general thesis that one

---

The Pygmalion experiment

In Rosenthal's exploration of the expectancy phenomenon among human subjects, all the children in an elementary school were administered a nonverbal test of intelligence, which was disguised as a test that would predict intellectual 'blooming'. There were eighteen classrooms in the school, three at each of the six grade levels. Within each grade level, the classrooms had been divided by the school according to ability: above average, average, and below average. Within each of the eighteen classrooms, approximately 20 per cent of the children were chosen at random to form the experimental group. Each teacher was given the names of the children from her class who were in the experimental situation. The teacher was told that the score attained by these children on the 'test for intellectual blooming' indicated that they would show remarkable gains in intellectual competence during the next eight months of school. The only difference between the experimental and control group children, then, was in the mind of the teacher.

At the end of the school year, eight months later, all the children were retested with the same intelligence test. The children from whom the teachers had been led to expect greater intellectual gain showed significantly greater increase in scores than did the children of the control group.

person's expectation can come to serve as a self-fulfilling prophecy for the behavior of another.

The implications for medical studies are fairly straightforward: the 'experimenter variable' (the term 'treatment behavior' has been used to characterize the social acts of those who profess to heal) cannot be ignored when planning bedside experiments.

USE OF PLACEBOS

A difficult question arises when a proposed intervention must be evaluated in a disorder for which there is no generally accepted standard treatment. Should a placebo, either an inert substance or a sham procedure, be prescribed for patients assigned to the untreated control category in a clinical trial? The dilemma is not easily resolved because the arguments are enmeshed quickly in a dense thicket of ethical issues.

Some public attitudes about the question were revealed during the years when attempts were made to reduce the risk of paralysis from poliomyelitis. In the 'double masked' trials of the 1950s to evaluate *prevention* of poliomyelitis, parents readily gave permission for enrollment of their children: 200 745 children received an injection of Salk vaccine and 201 229 received ineffective salt solution. On the other hand, there was considerable resistance to the conduct of a controlled trial challenging Sister Kenny's technique of hot packs which was used widely in this period for the early *treatment* of poliomyelitis.

A number of arguments can be mounted in favor of the use of placebos since inert materials and sham maneuvers may produce bodily effects that are quite striking and, many times, beneficial. There is, in fact, a placebo component in every clinical intervention and it is difficult to distinguish between specific and non-specific effects. Placebo responses may mimic effects produced by potent agents; the force of the phenomenon seems to derive from the ways in which patients interpret the therapeutic behavior of their doctors. The literal definition of the word placebo is 'I shall please.'

A remarkable example of the complex interactions in medical treatment was cited by Stewart Wolf of the University of Oklahoma. He told of a patient with long-standing and almost continuous asthma who obtained no relief from a series of drugs tried by the treating doctor. When an experimental drug with high promise of effectiveness became available, a supply was obtained by the doctor. The new drug relieved the asthmatic symptoms immediately; when it was stopped the asthma returned. The doctor substituted a placebo without the patient's knowledge; this failed to relieve symptoms. Shifts from new drug to placebo and back again were tried several times with consistent results in favor of the experimental agent. When the pharmaceutical company was approached for an additional supply, the doctor was amazed to learn that, because of worry about unjustified claims, the company had in this instance provided only a placebo preparation. The experience is a vivid reminder of the blurred distinction between treatment and non-treatment in placebo-control trials when doctors and patients are 'masked.'

Deliberate use of placebos has been a part of the healing art for centuries. Although there is tacit acceptance of the practice, it cannot be denied that patients may feel deceived and denigrated when sham treatments are prescribed solely to please them. ('Dummy,' the British term for a placebo is embarrassingly close in meaning to 'dolt' and 'stupid person'.) But the situation is arguably different in an organized effort to compare placebo and untested treatment. Here the protection of individual patients from unpredicted adverse effects is an uppermost goal and there is, I believe, ample justification for the tactic of placebo control.

The subject is controversial; pros and cons deserve a full debate whenever the use of a placebo is considered for a specific clinical trial. A compromise must be negotiated between the demands of objectivity, the obligation to uphold the dignity of participants, and the need for risk containment.

Multiple interventions

When compound treatments (multiple interventions applied concurrently or serially to the same patient) are tested, it is necessary to make simplifying assumptions to justify the approach. These premises are not badly strained when a single outcome-of-interest is assessed, but they are quickly overwhelmed when more than one result is evaluated.

Cross-over design

When the effects of treatments are temporary (that is, the effects during the first period do not carry over to the period of the next intervention) a cross-over design may be employed in which the patient serves as her/his own control. Comparison of three treatments (A, B, and C) can proceed by randomizing both the order of treatment and the entry of patients into the study:

	Treatment Periods		
	1	2	3
Patient 1	A	B	C
Patient 2	B	C	A
Patient 3	C	A	B

This 3×3 set of assignments is repeated so that at the end of the study there are an equal number of patients who have had treatments in each of treatment orders (for instance, A first, A second, A third, B first ...) The effect of order is now controlled and comparison between the three treatments can proceed.

Serial designs

In serial designs, the patient is exposed to different maneuvers according to a predetermined schedule, or successive treatments may be applied on a conditional basis.

Cross-over trials   The cross-over design is a scheduled plan that tests for transient effects of alternative treatments at different times in the same patient. The concept is attractive in that it increases the sensitivity of a trial by reducing between-subject variation in treatment comparisons. It must be assumed, however, that the patient returns completely to pre-treatment status with no carry-over effect between treatment. It should also be noted that a trial with an adequate number of patients for a sensitive comparison of treatments may be too small for detecting interaction between treatment and order.

Conditional treatments   In one form of serial treatments a second maneuver is applied *on condition* that the initial intervention has produced a specified result. The approach is used in the management of chronic illness and experimental trials that employ this design may mimic reality fairly closely.

For example, infants enrolled in an oxygen management trial who de-

---

Some biases in executing the experimental maneuver

Bogus control bias:

> When patients who are allocated to the experimental maneuver die or sicken before or during its administration and are omitted or reallocated to the control group, the favorable impression of the experimental maneuver is enhanced.

Co-intervention bias:

> In an experiment, when members of the experimental group receive treatments, attention or care (in addition to the experimental maneuver) which is not provided in equal amount to control, differences in outcome between experimental and control subjects may be spuriously attributed to the experimental maneuver.

Compliance bias:

> In experiments requiring patient adherence to therapy, issues of efficacy become confounded with those of compliance.

Contamination bias:

> In an experiment, when members of the control group inadvertently receive the experimental maneuver, the difference in outcomes between experimental and control patients may be systematically reduced.

Therapeutic personality bias:

> When treatment is not 'blind,' the therapist's convictions about efficacy may systematically influence both outcomes (positive personality) and their measurement (desire for positive results).

Withdrawal bias:

> Patients who are withdrawn from an experiment may differ systematically from those who remain.

(Described by Sackett)

velop early signs of RLF may then receive an additional maneuver purported to decrease the risk of blindness. The interpretation of the results of
the compound trial will be highly dependent upon the ability to establish a
uniform standard for the classification of 'early signs of RLF.' And care
must be taken to ensure that the outcomes are not distorted by the effects
of different oxygen treatments administered before the conditional maneuver was employed.

PROCEDURAL BIASES

The details of medical management are specified in the protocol of a clinical
trial. When systematic departures and unexpected complications in carrying
out the plan occur, they may overshadow other influences on outcome.

Co-intervention

The term 'co-intervention' refers to procedures (such as examinations, diagnostic tests, and auxillary treatments) that are performed on enrolled
patients. If these procedures are not performed with equal vigor on the
members of each group, confusing distortions may result.

In one survey of the relationship between RLF and the partial pressure
of oxygen in the blood of premature infants, the schedule for making these
measurements was not specified. When the results were inspected, there
appeared to have been a systematic bias toward more frequent measurement
of the oxygen status in babies at greater risk of developing RLF. The
resulting confusion from this defect in study design could not be unraveled
(with any confidence) by means of statistical adjustments.

Contamination

Inadvertent errors in the management of patients cannot be eliminated
entirely in the real world, and they occur, inevitably, in the best managed
trials. A patient may receive the same or a related treatment as the one
used in the comparison group, for example, and a decision must be made
about the disposition of this 'contamination' of the orderly trial. There is
a strong temptation to shift patients who inadvertently receive the alternative treatment to the 'correct' group on the logical grounds that this event
occurred 'by chance'. But a much stronger case can be made for retaining
the treated-by-error patients in the allocated group despite the error. In a
pragmatic trial, the report of the number of such errors provides a useful
bit of information because it provides a basis for estimating how often these
may be expected if the regimen is adopted for general use.

Similar problems arise with withdrawals from treatment and with failures
to comply with the prescribed course of treatment. All of these irregularities, again, provide important insights about the problems that will be

encountered when the results of the formal trial are translated into everyday actions.

Need for vigilance

Hugo Muench, of the Department of Biostatistics at the Harvard School of Public Health, became a legend in the field of biometry before his death in 1972. He proposed a number of droll 'laws' that provided considerable insight into the problems encountered in conducting clinical studies. A corollary of one of these is appropriate in summing up the intricacies in dealing with the issue of interventions. It reads: 'Anytime that things appear to be going well, you have overlooked something.'

Somewhat the same advice for those planning controlled trials was given by Donald Reid of the London School of Hygiene who recalled the words spoken by the White Queen to Alice in *Through the Looking Glass*: 'Consider what a great girl you are. Consider what a long way you've come today. Consider what o'clock it is. Consider anything ...' These words of caution have additional relevance at the stage in clinical trials when physician observers describe the outcomes of their interventions—the topic of the next two chapters.

6 Accurate observation

Doctors are trained to be careful observers. The teachings go back almost 2500 years to Hippocrates of Cos, who wrote:

It is the business of the physician to know, in the first place, things similar and things dissimilar; those connected with things most important, most easily known, and in anywise known; which are to be seen, touched, and heard; which are to be perceived in the sight, and the touch, and the hearing, and the nose, and the tongue, and the understanding; which are to be known by all the means we know other things.

Hippocrates on the appearance of the face in impending death

(Hippocratic Facies)
'... [the physician] should observe thus in acute diseases; first, the countenance of the patient, if it be like those of persons in health, and more so, if like itself, for this is the best of all; whereas the most opposite to it is the worst, such as the following; a sharp nose, hollow eyes, collapsed temples; the ears cold, contracted, and their lobes turned out; the skin about the forehead being rough, distended and parched; the color of the whole face being green, black, livid, or lead-colored. If the countenance be such at the commencement of the disease, and if this cannot be accounted for from the other symptoms, inquiry must be made whether the patient has long wanted sleep; whether his bowels have been very loose; and whether he has suffered from want of food; and if any of these causes be confessed to, the danger is to be reckoned so far less; it becomes obvious, in the course of a day and a night, whether or not the appearance of the countenance proceeded from these causes. But if none of these be said to exist, and if the symptoms do not subside in the aforesaid time, it is to be known for certain that death is at hand.'

The Hippocratic dicta led to the development of medical semeiology, the study of the signs and symptoms of disease. Medical practitioners began to compare, in detail, the condition of disease with that of health. In traumatic injuries, it became the practice of ancient surgeons to compare the injured part very carefully with its corresponding part on the opposite side. And 'all the means [by which] we know other things' referred to a new method of reasoning that replaced abstract speculation and the proclamation of oracles. The physician was encouraged to consider the logical consequences that follow from the information provided by the senses.

An original observation concerning the urine of a patient afflicted with diabetes as reported to the Medical Society of London in 1776 by Matthew Dobson

'Experiment V

After evaporating two quarts of urine to dryness by gentle heat, there remained a white cake, which was granulated and broke easily between the fingers. It smelled like brown sugar, neither could it from the taste be distinguished from sugar.'

Beginning with Hippocrates, attention was focused on the patient; the shift to accurate observation in medicine was as fundamental as the one that occurred when astrology was transformed into astronomy.

Doctor Joseph Bell's observations and deductions

In *The Man Who Was Sherlock Holmes,* Hardwick and Hardwick have written of the time when the young medical student, Arthur Conan Doyle, was appointed as out-patient clerk to his teacher, Doctor Bell. Sitting back in his chair, the surgeon quickly noted the peculiarities of the patients who were ushered into his room by Doyle. And he would address his clerk and a circle of medical students as follows: 'Gentlemen, I am not quite sure whether this man is a cork cutter or a slater. I observe a slight callus, or hardening, on one side of his forefinger, and a little thickening on the outside of this thumb, and that is a sure sign he is either one or the other.' Another case was simple: 'I see you're suffering from drink. You even carry a flask in the inside breast pocket of your coat.' A third patient listened open mouthed as Bell, after saying 'A cobbler, I see,' turned to his students and pointed out that the inside of the knee of the man's trousers was worn; that was where the man had rested the lapstone, a peculiarity only found in cobblers. One example of Bell's diagnoses impressed Doyle so much that he never forgot it:

'Well, my man, you've served in the army.'

'Aye, sir.'

'Not long discharged?'

'No, sir.'

'A Highland regiment?'

'Aye, sir.'

'A non-com. officer?'

'Aye, sir.'

'Stationed at Barbados?'

'Aye, sir.'

'You see, gentlemen,' explained Bell to his students, 'the man was a respectful man but he did not remove his hat. They do not in the army, but he would have learned civilian ways had he been long discharged. He had an air of authority and he is obviously Scottish. As to Barbados, his complaint is of elephantiasis, which is West Indian and not British.'

PHYSICIAN AS DETECTIVE

In the modern era, the name Sherlock Holmes has become the embodiment of the power of reasoning from observed facts. It is of interest that Holmes' creator, Arthur Conan Doyle, began his career as a physician and that the fictional detective was modeled after one of his teachers in medical school. The prototype, Doctor Joseph Bell, a Scottish surgeon at the Edinburgh Infirmary, explained to Doyle and to other medical students:

The precise and intelligent recognition and appreciation of minor differences is the real essential factor in all successful diagnosis ... Eyes and ears which can see and hear, memory to record at once and to recall at pleasure the impression of the senses, and an imagination capable of weaving a theory or piecing together a broken chain or unraveling a tangled clue, such are the implements of his trade to a successful diagnostician.

Although Doyle's stories celebrate the power of deductive reasoning, the detective's methods were not strictly deductive. Martin Gardner of *Scientific American* has noted that Holmes first tried to gather all the evidence that was relevant to the problem at hand, like a scientist trying to solve a mystery of nature. At times, he performed experiments to obtain fresh data. He then surveyed the total evidence in the light of his vast knowledge of crime, and of sciences relevant to crime, to arrive at the most probable hypothesis. Then the theory was further tested against new evidence, revised if need be, until the highly probable 'truth' emerged triumphantly.

The prepared mind

Notice, once more (p 15), that the sleuth's *initial* observations were, to use Popper's phrase, theory-impregnated. Holmes examined the evidence with a question in mind. The master detective's apotheosis, 'Joe' Bell, noted details about patients that entirely escaped the medical students (whose visual acuity was, very likely, much better than that of their older role model) because the experienced observer 'looked' with a prepared rather than an open mind. Moreover, the teacher used a limited number of 'off-the-shelf' theories; they were not constructed *de novo*. The inside of a trouser leg, frayed in a certain way, indicated to Bell the effect of a lap-held stone on which shoemakers beat leather, not the limitless possibilities that might be entertained by his students even after the physical clue was pointed out to them.

Pattern recognition methodology (used by detectives and by physicians) is, of course, a useful aid in everyday work but limitations do arise in the presence of novelty: we tend to see things we anticipate rather than the things that are there.

Preliminary notes on the character of Sherlock Holmes

In the first conception of the detective (who was to appear in the story *A Study in Scarlet*), Arthur Conan Doyle noted these words to himself: 'The Laws of Evidence.'

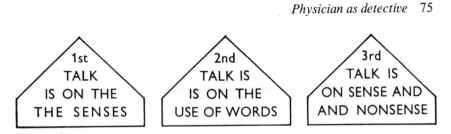

The lantern slide announcing the topics to be discussed in Asher's Lettsomian Lectures contains three printing errors.

Prefigured observation

The English clinician, Richard Asher, demonstrated our propensity to make what might be called prefigured observations and our unconscious dismissal of the anomalous. At the beginning of his Lettsomian Lectures delivered before the Medical Society of London in 1959, Asher projected a lantern slide announcing the topics to be covered in the series of talks. He intentionally 'planted' three gross printing errors in the announcement and later pointed out to the audience that only one person had caught the slips. A physician is both blessed and cursed by this suppressive mechanism, he noted, blessed when he detects an expected and significant pattern but cursed when significant irrelevancies are set aside without being appreciated.

The hidden man

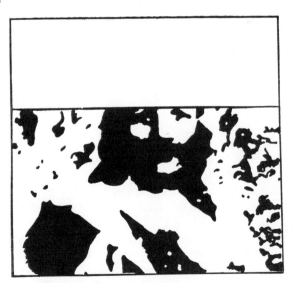

This incomplete picture demonstrates how a significant pattern remains hidden until the relevant and irrelevant features are sorted out. Once these are pointed out (see the 'solution' on p 76), it becomes almost impossible to *disregard* the face in this picture.

The recognition of significant patterns depends on past experiences and education, Asher argued, and he projected a figure of The Hidden Man (p 75) to demonstrate the point. Before the solution is 'taught', the pattern seems meaningless; after seeing the completed figure (below), the eye finds it almost impossible to return to its previous state, which was inexperienced, untutored, and, as a consequence, relatively unbiased.

'Solution' to the hidden man

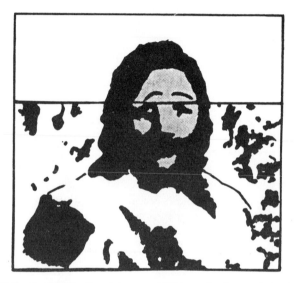

Additional details are added to the picture on p 75 to make the man's head and shoulders obvious. Now the pattern in the incomplete drawing cannot be erased from the 'seeing eye.'

PROPHECY ON TRIAL

It is unintentional 'within-observer' predilection, not conscious forgery, that is implied by the term 'observer's bias' in clinical trials involving conscientious physicians seeking fair appraisals of proposed treatments. The problem of biased observation must not be ignored; as I have emphasized repeatedly, observers should be 'masked' whenever it is technically possible and practical to do so.

On the surface, it may seem that scepticism is carried to unreasonable lengths when it is transferred from a concern with biasing effects of largely impersonal forces in the case of 'passive' observation to suspicions about the observer himself in 'active' observations. It may also appear frivolous to call for the judgment of an 'innocent' observer in the manner of a magician who must try to convince an audience of his supernatural powers.

> We travel like Ulysses to learn about the particolored world and its motley ways, but what we see is mostly controlled by patterns formed in our minds long before we took the first step.
>
> Robert M. Adams

These tactics seem out of place in a medical setting and when applied to matters of life and death. Indeed, both physicians and patients often resent the machinations; the precautions are perceived as an unworthy intrusion on a relationship of mutual trust. But when all is said and done in critical tests of hypotheses in medicine, acts of prophecy are on trial and prophets are simply not credible witnesses under these circumstances.

MEASUREMENT

When a proposition is subjected to a formal trial, the terms used in the measurement of the question to be addressed need to be specified. Before continuing, it will be useful to consider what is meant here by the word *measure*, since the concept of measurement is broadened in medicine to include more than the procedures used in physics to determine length, time, and mass. In the less precise operations ordinarily used in the social sciences and in medicine, several levels of measurement need to be distinguished.

Nominative classification

Nominal scales of measurement are used in the basic, descriptive stage of development of any scientific study. Persons or objects are classified with respect to a specified characteristic that can be identified reliably; but the characteristic does not have the property of size. For instance, when numbers are assigned to individuals according to country of birth (1. American, 2. Canadian, 3. French, ...) these numbers of a nominative scale cannot be ranked by size in a graded sequence. The aim is to sort individuals or other elements into defined categories; all individuals assigned to the category are equivalent in terms of the characteristic.

An axis of classification is particularly useful in medicine when collections of individuals are assembled who are alike with respect to some illness-related qualities. In the national RLF study, for example, the enrolled infants were sorted into 'single birth' or 'plural birth' classes; this identified groups of babies with strikingly different frequencies of RLF (twin, and other multiple births were affected three times more frequently than singletons). Classification is the *sine qua non* of all organized study of natural events; it is self-evident that all other levels of measurement, no matter how precise, involve categorization as a minimal operation. Moreover, if the

classes are exhaustive (for instance, 'single birth' and 'plural birth' categories include all new born infants) and mutually exclusive (each baby can
belong to only one class), we have the minimum requirements for numerical
analysis. Notice that the numbers used to count the frequency of individuals
assigned to the subclasses reflect the operation of enumeration, not the
operation of nominal scaling.

Exclusionary effect of categorization   Although nominative classification is
a powerful first step in organizing a body of information or an orderly
search for new information, it does have shortcomings. Whenever data are
summarized, certain information is inevitably lost. As a result, classification
limits and defines the range of possible conclusions that can be extracted
from the descriptive facts. The quip 'What you say is what you get' aptly
describes this constrictive effect of classification. Labeling bias stipulates the
level of entry into an inquiry, and such effects cannot be completely eliminated by refined definitions. The nominalists are quite correct when they
maintain that to define *is* to leave out. It must be recognized that each
summarizing process is an abstraction which imposes limitations, and the
implications that flow from the level of abstraction used must not be
ignored.

Problem-specific classification   In recent years, classification of infants by
birthweight *and* by functional indicators of development has provided considerable insight into problems that were blurred previously, but the categories are still quite non-specific. RLF occurs almost exclusively in infants
with incomplete development of the blood vessels of the retina; thus, an
elementary 'one–zero' scale for the 'presence' or 'absence' of an immature
network of retinal vessels would be a useful first step in a problem-specific
classification of babies for RLF studies. (This variety of unranked scale is
called 'existential'.) Unfortunately, technical barriers make it impractical to
use the criterion in the smallest babies as the normally clear, forward portion of the eye—the vitreous—is hazy in the first days of life and this makes
it difficult to inspect the retinal layer which lies behind it, until the infants
are one to two weeks old.
   Practical difficulties of this kind are common in medicine: the realities
must be acknowledged, but they are also quite challenging. Formal investigations often provide an opportunity for the development of improved
nominal scales for the highly relevant but vaguely defined information collected by observation at the bedside. The physician observer is the 'measuring instrument' and the object is to devise classifications that are directly
related to clinical problems.

Ordinal succession

The level of measurement is raised when we can make use of the concept of numbered succession in the form of ordinal scales. This refinement becomes possible when the magnitude of qualities can be compared. If we can place individuals in an ordered succession, along a continuous scale of size, there will be 'ties' and 'near ties' who resemble one another very closely and they may be assigned to mutually exclusive classes. But the between-class distinctions are now quantified. This kind of measurement is higher than the primary level; for, in addition to the nominative operation, the categories can be ranked in a size-determined order.

In RLF, the blood vessels of the retina undergo changes that can be detected with an ophthalmoscope. The aberrations begin when infants are several weeks old and progress over a period of weeks and months; the changes may regress completely, go on to leave scars in the eye, or advance to complete blindness. Stages of increasing severity were classified (in 1953) into ten grades (stages I to V for the early blood vessel changes and a set of five grades for the late scarring lesions). These ordinal scales were very useful in making semiquantitative statements about RLF when the disorder was occurring in epidemic frequency.

The ordinal level of measurement does not supply any information about the size of differences between the grades of the continuum. We can only declare (in RLF) that the larger numbers represent an increased intensity of the process, but we cannot express the relationships in familiar mathematical terms. Addition or subtraction is possible, but only in a restricted sense. For instance, if RLF activity (early blood vessel changes) is represented by distance along a continuum:

Normal	I	II		III	IV	V

we can say that the distance $I-V = I-II + II-III + III-IV + IV-V$, but we cannot make valid statements about the relationships between distances I–II and II–III ... IV–V.

When we translate order relationships with indeterminate intervals into arithmetic operations, we cannot justify the use of the ordinary processes of addition, subtraction, multiplication, and division. Nonetheless, the fact that we can make comparisons such as 'greater than' and 'less than' represents a step up from the lower scale of measurement.

Scores Dimensional appraisal of the physical signs and subjective symptoms of illness may be expressed in the form of scores. Severity or intensity, for instance, are ranked according to specified rules for assigning one, and only one, number on an ordinal scale of values. The score is developed by choosing a number of items that are thought to be related to the quality that is characterized and then selecting, by trial, the elements that are consistent in the way they order patients.

Although relatively few of these scalar methods have been used in medicine, there is no logical reason for avoiding such aids to the organization of the rich store of observations about the uniquely human aspects of illness.

Interval and ratio scales

The next levels in the hierarchy of measurements (interval and ratio scales) require the use of standard units (such as meters, kilograms, and degrees of temperature) to express quantity. A distinction is made between an interval system in which a numbered scale of equal units begins at an arbitrary zero and a ratio system of numbers in which zero indicates absence of a measured property. An interval scale allows us to determine only that two objects differ by a certain amount of the property. The highest scale of measurement permits statements about the ratios that obtain between the measured properties.

For example, the Celsius system of temperature measurement is an interval scale (0°C is arbitrarily set at the freezing point of water); as a result we can determine, say, that $50°C - 25°C = 25°C$, but $50°C \div 25°C \neq 2$; we are not justified in declaring that 50°C is twice as warm as 25°C. Temperature measured in the Kelvin system is a ratio scale (O°K, absolute zero, is the temperature at which molecules stop moving and there is literally 'no heat'); here differences *and* ratios reflect the real world. There are no restrictions on arithmetic operations carried out on numbers obtained in ratio scale measurements.

Valid arithmetic

Notice that each level of measurement has distinct properties, and that the levels themselves form a cumulative scale. An ordinal scale has all the characteristics of a nominal scale plus ordinality. An interval scale has all the qualities of both lower scales plus a unit of measurement, and a ratio scale, representing the highest level, has a unit of measurement and a meaningful zero. It is logical to drop back one or more levels if necessary in the course of analyzing data, but it is quite illogical to move up the hierarchy if the underlying assumptions necessary to perform arithmetic operations have not been satisfied.

There are no inherent safeguards that prevent us, for example, from using numbers obtained in ordinal measurements for a calculation which requires a higher scale (such as calculating the arithmetic mean of the stages of RLF); only reasoning back to the nature of the measurement will prevent such errors. The appropriate use of measurement, like the correct use of language, depends entirely on the user.

Addition

A man begging for money summarized his plight on a sign next to his tin cup. It read:

Wars	2
Legs	1
Wives	2
Children	4
Bankruptcies	2
Total	11

ACCURACY IN MEASUREMENT

There are no units of measure for many of the signs and symptoms that constitute the raw knowledge of bedside medicine. As a result, laboratory measurements that can be expressed by interval and ratio scale numbers are often collected as proxies for ordinal or nominal information in the hope of reducing subjective influences on observations.

Observer error

There is a mistaken belief that rigor and precision are associated only with the higher levels of measurement. An uncritical sense of confidence seems to develop when measurements are made by others using instruments at some distance from the bedside. I find it interesting that the observers who are entirely dependent on instruments to make measurements on the objects farthest removed from our direct sense experience, the astronomers, were the first to become curious about the personal element in instrumental errors of measurement.

Kinnebrook's defect In August 1795, Maskelyne, the royal astronomer at the Greenwich Observatory, found that his assistant, Kinnebrook, was recording the movements of stars across the sky about a half-second 'too slow' (when compared with Maskelyne's records). He was convinced that all through 1794 there had been no discrepancy. Maskelyne cautioned Kinnebrook about the 'error'; nevertheless, it increased during the succeeding months until, in January 1796, it had become about eight tenths of a second. At this point, Maskelyne dismissed his assistant.

The error was serious; the calibration of the Greenwich clock, the standard of time on which many other calculations were made, depended upon these stellar transit speeds. (They were made by an 'eye and ear' method: the field of a telescope was divided by parallel crosswires in the reticle; the observational problem consisted of noting, to one tenth of a second from the audible beats of a clock, the time at which a given star crossed a given wire.) Kinnebrook's error of eight tenths of a second was a relatively large one and seemed to justify Maskelyne's conclusion that the man had fallen 'into some irregular and confused method of his own'.

The incident was recorded in the pages of *Astronomical Observations at Greenwich*, and would have passed into oblivion had it not come to the attention of an astronomer at Königsberg, named Bessel, some twenty years later. The experience struck him as odd and he considered the possibility that the errors were not willful. It seemed to Bessel that Kinnebrook, when informed of his 'error', must have tried to correct it. The failure to succeed, he thought, might mean the error was involuntary. Bessel set out to study the observations of stellar transits made by a number of senior astronomers. Differences in observation, he discovered, were the rule, not the exception.

'Personal equation' of observers A good deal of interest in the problem was generated by these findings and efforts were made to 'calibrate the observer' in the hope of correcting for the deviations of observation. In the 1840s, the practice of measuring the 'personal equation', as it came to be called, became common among astronomers. In addition to determining the 'absolute' personal equation for each observer, the 'personalities' of the eye, of the ear, and of touch were calculated. The prevailing notion was that these variations between observers were related only to physiological differences (and were unique for each astronomer), but, by the 1870s, it slowly became clear that there were psychological variants that accounted for the personal variability in observations.

Confirmation bias Contemporary research on the measurement performance of scientists has demonstrated that observer errors tend to produce results which lean in the direction of the observer's hypothesis. In one set of studies, recording errors by experimenters in behavioral research were not frequent (1 per cent of over 20 000 observations), but when the errors did occur, more than two thirds of the time they were in the direction of the recorder's hypothesis. Laboratory workers, looking for hours at a pointer on a scale or digital displays, develop subconscious ideas, it seems, as to the 'proper behavior' of the inanimate devices.

Properties of sets of measurements

The third replicate Readings in a time sequence often reveal a type of expectancy bias and an effort must be made to ensure that repeat measurements are truly independent. The issue arises, for example, when three successive measurements of a single object are made to calculate the mean. If the last value does not fall in the range between the first two, there is a temptation to replace it with a 'better' measurement. Many years ago, W.J. Youden of the National Bureau of Standards pointed out that chance

The behavior of sets of measurements

Consider a set of three measurements which are made sequentially, Youden has said. After the first two are made, how often will the third measurement fall between the two? (No assumption needs to be made that the measurements follow a symmetrical distribution.) Indicate on a scale the position of three measurements, A, B, and C:

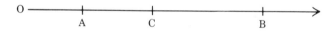

Here C does lie between A and B, but the three measurements might have fallen in any one of six ranked orders in which they can be arranged:

Rank order	1	2	3
	A	C	B*
	A	B	C
	B	A	C
	B	C	A*
	C	A	B
	C	B	A

* These are the only two, out of six equally likely sequences, that bring C between A and B

Thus, it follows that one third of the sets of measurements will be such that the third measurement falls between those already made. Two times out of three, in the long run, the third measurement will be smaller than both or larger than both the first pair. The general formula for this property of data reads: If $(n-1)$ measurments are followed by an nth measurement, the chance that this measurement falls between the smallest and the largest of the $(n-1)$ measurements is $(n-2)/n$. For example, in sets of ten measurements, once out of five times, the tenth measurement will be either smaller or larger than the other nine.

variation of independent measurements is worth considering when these are made in sets.

The behavior of sets of three measurements is such that the third measurement falls between the two already made only one third of the time, in the long run. This property of data cannot be changed by anything the observer can do, since it results from the action of the goddess of fortune.

Size of the outlying replicate School courses in quantitative chemical analysis often require that students turn in duplicate analytic results. The grade for the exercise depends in part on how well the average of the two determinations agrees with the value ascribed to the material and, in part, on how well the two agree with each other. Students commonly perform three 'runs' and turn in the pair showing the best agreement. Studies of the behavior of measurements, however, indicate that the dispersion of the average of selected pairs is greater than that exhibited by unselected duplicates. The properties of sets of three measurements are such that it appears

The 'outlying' value in sets of three measurements

When a set of three measurements is made, it frequently happens that two are in close agreement and the third lies considerably removed from the pair. There is a strong temptation to discard the outlying value, on the basis of an intuitive feeling that a blunder accounts for the apparent discrepancy. Unless there is some conception of the ways three measurements may distribute themselves when there is nothing whatsoever wrong with any of them, a judgment as to whether or not a 'slip' has been made is almost certain to err in discarding good values. Consider again, Youden argued, the three measurements marked off on a linear scale; this time the distances between them are denoted as d and D:

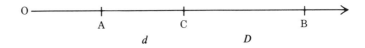

It has been shown that the interval D is at least four times as large as d more than a third of the time, and it is ten or more times as large as d in 15.7 per cent of sets of three measurements. Values of the ratio D/d exceed 32.57 once in twenty times according to studies conducted at the National Bureau of Standards. Thus, if there is no knowledge about the dispersion of values, there is little justification for discarding the remote value unless it is removed from the closest pair by an amount some thirty times the difference between the measurements constituting the closest pair.

unwise to discard an 'outlying' value unless it is removed from the closest pair by an amount some thirty times the difference between the close-lying pair.

Terminology

Terms to distinguish the kinds of errors encountered in observations are used rather loosely. To reduce confusion, it is helpful to define the words when they are used in reports of medical studies.

The term *accuracy* is often used to indicate the degree of agreement between an observation and its true value; the latter can be determined when refined methods of measurement are available. Similarly, measurements are said to be *unbiased* if they do not systematically overstate or understate the true value of a characteristic. On the other hand, *precision* (*reliability* and *consistency*) measures the extent to which a series of observations agree with one another—the repeatability of the results of measurement.

The distinction between accuracy (lack of bias) and precision (reliability, consistency) is of importance in clinical medicine, where there is often preoccupation with repeatability because there is no objective method of measuring the 'true' value. A set of bedside observations can be inaccurate yet quite precise. Agreement between observers, and in repeated observations by the same observer, gives no assurance of accuracy.

> Immersion in water makes the straight seem bent: but reason thus confused by false appearances is beautifully restored by measuring, numbering and weighing: these drive vague notions of greater or less or more or heavier right out of the minds of the surveyor, the computer, and the clerk of the scales. Surely it is the better part of thought that relies on measurement and calculation.
>
> Socrates

Validity of measurement tends to connote accuracy, but, as with the latter term, the exact meaning is fuzzy when there is no accepted outside standard for comparison. For example, validity is often defined as the extent to which an observer measures what he or she claims to measure. The definition is suspended in thin air if the claim is described in terms of the measure: 'intelligence is what intelligence tests measure.' I will explore these problems further in the next chapter.

Observations of natural events proceed, it has been said, with a 'mixture of clear logic and unwritten superstition'. And yet the replacement of hunches and guesses in medicine with measurements of the course of disease and the effects of treatment is secure. Measurement is the fibre of modern medicine.

7 The event of interest

In modern laboratory experiments, the efforts to reproduce predicted outcome events reliably are largely successful. The doubts that I mentioned in the last chapter need to be put into perspective. Accuracy in laboratory measurements has improved to the point that experimental errors in many procedures are regarded as merely nuisances that can be controlled by careful attention to detail. And, as I have suggested, such technical capability often leads to a dilemma when we must choose an outcome criterion in a pragmatic clinical trial. Should we record what we can measure with minimum error or measure what we think is directly relevant with the highest accuracy possible? In medicine, we often find ourselves in the position of the drunk who dropped his key in a dark hallway and was observed looking for it under the street lamppost: 'The light is better here,' he explained.

SURROGATE OUTCOME

Proxy outcome-events are often chosen in medical trials because of technical limitations, the impracticality of prolonged observation, and also because of moral restraints.

Survival as an outcome indicator

Concerns about mixed end results of modern care of premature infants have grown in recent years as life-support methods have become more intensive. A prominent question is, Have recently introduced, highly developed techniques of diagnosis and treatment improved the outlook for these small babies? The ongoing uncertainty has not been resolved, since much of the difficulty centers around the matter of deciding what outcome events should be chosen as measures of 'improved outlook.'

For many years the efforts to better the prospects for premature babies were measured by a decrease in neonatal mortality rate (deaths during the first 28 days of life among liveborn infants weighing less than 2.5 kilograms). Surveys in the 1960s, however, indicated that the relationship be-

Death and survival-with-handicap in small premature infants

An alternate-assignments trial of intensive care

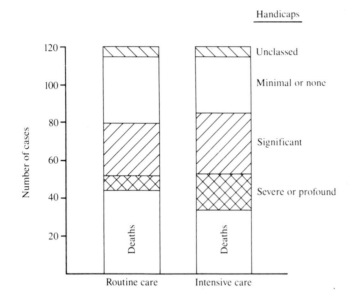

Frequency of death and handicap at 8 years of age among 238 prematurely born children (birthweight 1–1.5 kilograms) who had been assigned, by Kitchen and co-workers, to routine or intensive neonatal care on an alternating basis on arrival in the hospital. Infants with gross abnormalities at birth were not enrolled in the trial. Severe or profound handicaps included major sensory, intellectual, and motor disabilities; significant handicaps included motor incoordination, epilepsy, and serious visual problems. (Redrawn from the figure of Kitchen and co-workers.)

tween rapidly falling mortality rate among the smallest neonates and the risk of survival with major handicap was complex.

An alternate-assignment clinical trial to compare the results of routine versus intensive care of premature infants was conducted by W.H. Kitchen and co-workers of the University of Melbourne between 1966 and 1970. The Australian researchers observed that an increased survival attributable to vigorous techniques of treatment may have been achieved at the expense of an increased number of severely handicapped children. Surveys conducted in the 1970s suggested that both mortality and the frequency of m'jor handicap have decreased, but the controversial issue about the full impact of modern life-support techniques in the management of very small babies has not been subjected to further testing with concurrent controls. Ethical conflicts make it virtually impossible to conduct rigorous tests of the questions about opposing end points—in this case, death versus disability—of different policies of treatment.

A conflict of perspectives   When there is a conflict in outcomes, which event of interest is appropriate in a planned trial? It is impossible to avoid a value-oriented point of view. It happens, not infrequently, that the perspective of the medical profession differs from that of the community at large or from specific groups in a plural society.

Some of the misunderstanding about medicine's mission becomes evident when we examine the word 'lifesaving' as used to describe a medical procedure. The idea of 'saving lives' is deeply ingrained in the medical thinking (it is uncomfortably close to the evangelist's conception of 'saving souls'). But death is inevitable; it can merely be postponed, even by the most successful treatments.

Quality of life as an outcome indicator

The outcome of interest to each individual and to the community at large is life prolongation, rather than death. The former 'event' is difficult to measure. It is not a discrete function, it is a continuous variable with a concrete temporal dimension and innumerable value-defined qualities. In addition to short-term considerations, there are long-term effects of medical interventions that must be taken into account.

In a review of assessments in studies of surgical treatments John P. Gilbert and associates of Harvard University found most concern with immediate outcomes. Information about the quality of life of patients was

---

Euphranor: Tell me, Alciphron, can you discern the doors, window and battlements of that same castle?

Alciphron: I cannot. At this distance it seems only a small round tower.

Euphranor: But I, who have been in it, know that it is no small round tower, but a large square building with battlements and turrets, which it seems you do not see.

Alciphron: What will you infer from thence?

Euphranor: I would infer that the very object which you strictly and properly perceive by sight is not that thing which is several miles distant.

Alciphron: Why so?

Euphranor: Because a little round object is one thing, and a great square object is another. Is it not so? ... Is it not plain, therefore, that ... the castle, *which you see there* [is not that] real one which you suppose exists at a distance?

Bishop George Berkeley

usually missing. For proper evaluation of alternative surgical treatments, the reviewers argued, there is a need to assess the patient's residual symptoms, state of restored health, feeling of well-being, limitations, new or restored capabilities, and responses to these advantages or disadvantages. In the case of infants and children, for example, the immediate consequences of treatments are often dwarfed by those that become manifest during the long lifetime ahead.

Limitations of short-term studies   The important weaknesses of studies of short-term effects of treatments are self-evident, but it is difficult to devise stronger approaches. The passage of time introduces confounding influences and imposes major impediments. It must be supposed, for example, that long-term outcomes are related to an early intervention, not to some intervening influences. Enormous organizational efforts are required to sustain follow-up study of highly mobile modern populations, and even the limited life span of investigators conspires against the best laid plans to conduct prolonged observations. Finally, the discovery of an unexpected outcome after years of observation, marks the beginning, not the end, of investigation.

Hippocrates was well aware of the constrictions imposed by time in medical study. The opening passage in his first book of *Aphorisms* notes: 'Life is short and Art long; the occasion fleeting; experience fallacious, and judgment difficult.'

ACCOUNTING OF TIME-RELATED EVENTS

The 'flight of time'—duration of various states and timing of events—needs to be examined in considerable detail so that the limitations of a circumscribed clinical trial are clearly in view.

The 'trial time' of each patient

A number of complexities are introduced when patients are recruited over a designated period of time (they are rarely available all at once). In changing proportions over the course of a study, the enrolled population normally consists of individuals who have completed treatment, others who are undergoing treatment, and newly enrolled patients who are about to be treated. The duration of a study may be a fixed interval marked off by the calendar or a span of time that is determined by enrollment of a specified number of individuals.

The dizzying array of time designations is best expressed in terms of a basic unit, the trial time, determined for each patient. This interval of time begins at the moment of assignment-by-lot to a treatment category and

The life-table method of expressing outcome

Abbreviated version

A life-table is an efficient accounting form for summarizing the survival experience of an at-risk population over a specified period of time (newborn infants in the first week of life, for instance). For this approach, the number of individuals who were alive at the beginning of a specific age interval (l_x) and the number who died during that interval (d_x) are set out as follows:

l_x	226	85	62	51	47	46	44
d_x	141	23	11	4	1	2	1
p_x	0.38	0.73	0.82	0.92	0.98	0.96	0.98

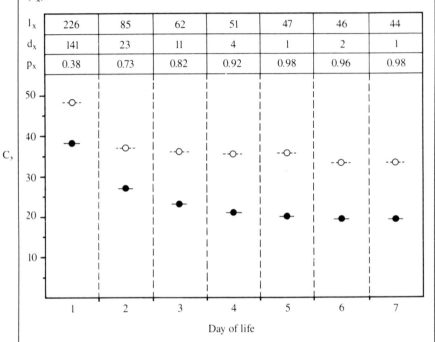

Day of life

The table indicates the survivorship of 226 male infants (birthweight ≤ 1.5 kilograms born during the years of oxygen curtailment, 1955–7) in the first 7 days of life. On the first day of life there were 141 deaths; thus the survival rate for this age interval is:

$$p_1 = 1 - \left(\frac{d_1}{l_1}\right) = 1 - \left(\frac{141}{226}\right) = 0.38, \text{ the } observed \ survival \ rate$$

and on day 2 there were 23 deaths (d_2) among $226 - 141 = 85$ survivors (l_2) thus,

$$p_2 = 1 - \left(\frac{23}{85}\right) = 0.73$$

$p_3 \ldots p_7$ are calculated similarly

These observed rates provide a rough estimate of the probability of survival for each of the days after birth. We may then argue that the way to live 7 days after birth is to be alive for 6 days and then live one more day. Thus, the probablity of living 7 days is the probability of living 6 days multiplied by the chance of surviving day 7:

$$C_1 \times C_2 \times C_3 \ldots \times C_7$$

where,

C_1 is the chance of surviving at least one day after birth
C_2 is the chance of surviving a second day *after* surviving the first day of life
$C_3 \ldots C_7$

The true values for these cumulative probabilities (Cs) are unknown, but we may estimate any one (C_7, for example) by calculating the product of the *observed* survival rates:

$$C_7 = p_1 \times p_2 \dots p_7 = 0.38 \times 0.73 \dots \times 0.98 = 0.19$$

The life-table estimates of C_1 through C_7 for males are plotted in the graph $-\bullet-$ (The values for females are plotted for contrast $-\bigcirc-$; the base numbers are not shown.)

The life-table approach is a useful way to express survival after treatment (trial time, not age, is used for this application). Importantly, it draws attention to the issue of duration of exposure to risk and durations of observations.

ends with the occurrence of an event of interest (such as time of death, disappearance or appearance of an arbitrary manifestation).

In most medical trials, all patients do not experience the event of interest; the trial time runs to the pre-designated termination of the period of observations. Inevitably, there are incomplete observations because enrollment terminates on an agreed upon date before the latest participants have completed the prescribed period of observation, because patients are withdrawn or otherwise default, and because patients fail to return for follow-up in a long-term study. These unequal time durations need to be accounted for in some orderly fashion.

Life-table accounting of events

The life-table method of 'bookkeeping' (used to make actuarial calculations) provides a very useful solution to the maddening time-related problems of accountancy in medical trials.

The basic idea behind the life-table approach to the expression of event rates is found in the following statement: to survive a whole week, a patient must survive each of the 7 days comprising it. Although seemingly trivial, this simple tautology is the key to an efficient scheme for expressing outcome. For example, among 439 very small babies born over a three-year period (1955–7), only 116 survived the first week of life: 44 of 226 males (19 per cent) and almost twice that proportion among females, 72 of 213 (33 per cent). This overall summary provides no estimation of the gradations of risks in the two sexes that occurred from birth through the seventh day. But they are clearly expressed by the use of life-table bookkeeping to record the experience.

We begin with 226 boys at birth, for instance, and record the losses incurred by this cohort on each day of life. During the age interval 0–24 hours (day 1) there were 141 deaths, leaving 85 who were available to undertake the risks of the second day. Of these, 23 succumbed on day 2; and the decimations continued until there were 44 boys left to face the risks of the seventh day of life. Daily outcome rates are now calculated and these are used to calculate estimates of cumulative probabilities in actuarial fashion.

The initial cohort of patients and the number alive at the beginning of each age interval have been compared rudely to the contenders in each round of a steeplechase. Only the entrants who are present at the start of a round provide useful information about the risk of the up-coming circuit. And an estimate of the probability of completing the race is provided only by riders who successfully complete each round.

Life-tables may be elaborated to account for latecomers and withdrawals whose contribution to the estimates of risk is adjusted for curtailed periods and durations of exposure and observation. Feinstein has pointed out that the 'pat' solutions of the life-table must not be accepted uncritically. For example, the assumption that the age of infants transferred from various hospitals is the most important risk characteristic to be considered, should not go unchallenged. And the reasons for withdrawal may be more relevant than the age of withdrawal. Nevertheless, the life-table format makes it relatively easy for an 'auditor' to spot time-related problems of account-ability which remain hidden in other forms of documenting outcomes in comparative trials.

CONFIRMING CRITERIA FOR OUTCOMES

Four requirements have been proposed for the characteristics of observa-tions used to decide that an event of interest has, in fact, taken place. Individual diagnostic criteria or tests that are used in medical trials should be reproducible, discriminatory, accurate, and as simple as possible.

Reproducibility of confirming observations

The reproducibility (yet another term for precision, p 84) of confirming observations depends on the inherent consistency of the measurement or test in *everyday* circumstances, the constancy of the object or quality that is measured, and the ability of the observer to interpret and record what he or she has measured. Some of the general sources of variation in observa-tions were discussed in Chapter 6. Here I wish to emphasize the variation in phenomena as they take place at the bedside.

With few exceptions, the characteristics of patients change with time, many manifestations fluctuate (regularly and irregularly), and the variation in states is made to appear even greater when the conditions are measured indirectly by signs determined on physical examination. Thus, it is the pattern of dispersion of the diagnostic observations that is the replication sought in sets of clinical observations.

Observer error versus observer variation   It is useful to distinguish between two kinds of misclassification made by observers. As we have seen (p 81), *observer error* refers to the mistakes that can be demonstrated either by

Cusum plot method of expressing trends

Serial measurements of characteristics which fluctuate widely (like body temperature in febrile states) are difficult to summarize, and trends are often obscured because of the scatter of values. The plotting of cumulative sums ('cusums') is a useful method of transforming unruly numbers.

The first step is the selection of a reference value, such as the approximate mean of the original data points. In the example given by Herbert Wohl of the University of California (serial body temperatures in a patient with a serious blood disorder),

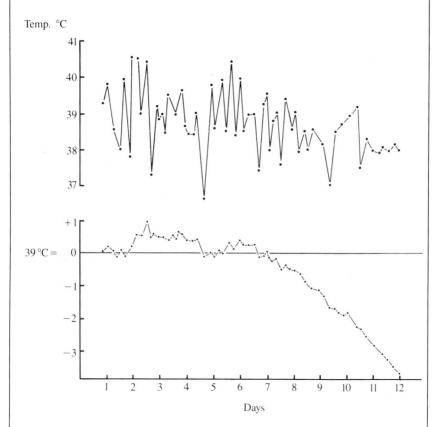

the plot in the upper panel indicates the observed fluctuations. Choosing 39°C as a reference point, it is subtracted from each data point in succession. Any remainder is added algebraically to the previous sum. If the temperature remained at exactly 39°, the plot would remain at the reference-zero line.

The cusum values are plotted in the lower panel and the transformed scale clearly demonstrates a downward sloping line beginning on day 8 (the trend is difficult to make out in the conventional fever chart in the upper panel). A change in slope represents a change in mean value; the distance from the reference value is disregarded—only a change in slope matters. The greater the change in slope, the greater the change in mean.

majority opinion of a number of observers, by the same evaluator at a subsequent re-examination, or by an independent criterion of assessment.

On the other hand, disagreement between observers or inconsistent evaluations by the same observer may not stem entirely from perceptual error. *Observer variation* may be due to the fact that a significant number of observations fall close to the boundary between categories. For example, in an effort to improve the reliability of observations, two or more ophthalmologists may conduct independent examinations of the eyes of premature infants. When there is disagreement, the disputed interior of the eye is re-examined and discussed until agreement is reached. This may simply result in deference to the most experienced or most domineering observer. Forced agreement may obliterate the very fact that the verdict on certain examinations *is* doubtful. When categorical judgments are made concerning a process that is continuous in nature, the fact that disagreements occur most often near a boundary should suggest the need for a finer scale of measurement.

Standardization of observations   Observer error and variability may be reduced by efforts to 'tune' the skills of observers. This is accomplished by practice sessions in preparation for formal studies; it is particularly useful in preparing for a collaborative study that will involve observers in different hospitals.

A descriptive 'standard' is also a helpful device for improving the precision of observations in clinical trials. For example, a verbal description and set of drawings of the appearance of the retina at each of the stages of RLF was used in the national study of this disorder in an effort to achieve reproducibility of diagnoses from one institution to the next.

The Rumpelstiltskin effect

Richard Asher pointed out the power of words in medicine: however uninformative the name of his or her illness may be, a patient feels the foe is partially vanquished once the name is disclosed. A typical exchange sounds like this:

'I seem to have an inflamed tongue, doctor. Will you have a look at it?'

'Ah, yes. You've got glossitis.'

'Thank you, doctor. It's all right now that I know what it is.'

The phenomenon is called the Rumpelstiltskin Effect, after the nursery story of the miller's daughter who got into the clutches of a dwarf. Having pretended she could spin straw into gold, she was put to the test, and she was in despair until the little man came and did it for her. The dwarf then blackmailed the unfortunate girl and would only relinquish his claims if she could guess his name. She managed to get hold of his name, finally, by a trick and was freed.

But no wonder the dwarf was confident that he could not be undone: Rumpelstiltskin was the kind of name unlikely to occur to a nicely brought up maiden; it means 'crinkly foreskin'.

Glossary of terms It is also important to recognize problems that arise with terminology in formal studies. Everyday definitions of medical terms are often imprecise; additionally, the bestowal of a name on a concept, whether real or imaginary, may bring it into clinical existence. It is useful to prepare a glossary as an appendix to the protocol, providing a list of terms that will be used in the trial and definitions to serve as the common standard.

Discrimination and accuracy of diagnoses

The characteristics of discrimination and accuracy as applied to confirming observations in clinical trials refer to the correct sorting in a diagnostic classification (the nominal and ordinal operations of measurement).

Ideal observations and tests would place all the unaffected in one class and all affected in their correct positions in the remaining class or classes. In practice, lack of discrimination may result from poor correlation between the degree of abnormality as shown by test and the severity of the target condition in fact. For example, the eye changes (that occur in a relatively small proportion of infants exposed to supplemental oxygen) may turn out to be highly inaccurate criteria for separating oxygen-affected and un-affected babies if, say, late appearing neurological signs should indicate that the frequency of oxygen-induced damage to the brain is higher than has been appreciated.

Expressing the accuracy of diagnostic tests

Result of a test	Confirmed* status of a condition	
	Present	Absent
Positive	a	b
Negative	c	d

'True-positive' ratio $= a/a+c$
'True-negative' ratio $= d/b+d$

The proportion of patients correctly classified as 'positive', (a), among a group who are affected by a disorder, ($a+c$), reflects the *sensitivity* of a diagnostic test. Similarly, the fraction of 'true-negatives', (d), among those free of the disorder, ($b+d$), is a measure of the *specificity* of the test.

These estimates are relevant only to the particular experience reported since the values are dependent upon the proportion of abnormals in a given sample. Moreover, the labels 'sensitivity' and 'specificity' determined in this way should not be regarded as inherent properties of the test or observation. (The estimates of predictive accuracy, i.e. $a/a+b$ and $d/c+d$, must be interpreted with considerable caution.)

* Confirmation by some independent criterion.

Evaluation of accuracy   When there is an independent (and unequivocal) method of confirming the occurrence of an event of interest, the calculation of 'true-positive' and 'true-negative' ratios of observations provides a limited basis for describing their accuracy. These estimates cannot be extended (with any assurance) beyond the particular experience under study, but they do provide a method of comparing different diagnostic criteria for the same event and between-observer differences in diagnoses.

Simple criteria of outcome

Finally, the requirement of simplicity of differential criteria takes into account the practical matters of patient comfort, time, and expense in carrying out studies involving suffering human beings. Careful consideration must be given to the cost, in these practical terms, whenever elaborate tests and observations are proposed in exchange for relatively small gains in discrimination.

At every step in the planning of studies that require people to enroll in a regimented program, we must return to the questions concerning external relevance: To whom are the results of the study meant to apply? At the event-of-interest step we must ask, Are the diagnostic criteria practical for everyday application? The pros and cons as seen from a community-wide perspective must be weighed before deciding on the observations and tests that are to be used in a bedside trial.

TARGET EVENTS

How many target events may be 'lined up in a row' in a focused clinical trial? Common sense and good citizenship require that we try to obtain as much firm evidence as possible when we undertake an exercise that places so many demands on the participants and on the community's resources. But how can these stipulations be met, given the actions of the 'inconstant, dangerous, and delicately balanced' goddess of fortune? (As the number of end-points increases, the likelihood of chance associations *must* rise.)

The dilemma can be resolved if we make a clear distinction between three kinds of targets: a 'called shot', several 'practice targets', and lastly, unexpected 'hits'. If we are to use the logic of chance as a guide to the interpretation of the occurrence of observed events, we are forced to return to the aim of the study: the results must be examined in the context of the pre-trial questions and the details of the experimental design.

Primary event of interest

The primary target event is the outcome that is defined in terms which relate to the specific question posed before the trial begins. (In the national RLF trial, the primary outcome of interest was the appearance of scarring eye changes during a trial time that concluded when each infant reached the age of $2\frac{1}{2}$ months.) It is the number of such outcome events that determines the dimensions of the trial, and it is the prediction about these numbers that is put to a severe test. (The proportional proposition that risked refutation in the RLF trial stated that curtailed oxygen management was expected to reduce the frequency of the scarring form of RLF in enrolled babies from a little over 10 per cent to about 2 per cent or less).

> Since the principle of life in animals is a force which is ever active, which is constantly endeavoring to overcome obstacles, and since nature when left to its own devices cures many diseases by itself, it follows that when a remedy is applied, it is infinitely difficult to determine what effects are due to nature and what to the remedy. The result presents itself to the wise man merely as a greater or lesser probability, and that probability can be converted into certainty only by a large number of facts of the same kind.
>
> Lavoisier (1784)

Total number of primary events Comparative trials are relatively insensitive to fairly substantial true differences between treatments because chance variations in outcomes between groups of patients tend to be quite large. The fluctuations in the usual small-scale trial may either obscure true differences or excite false interest in a new intervention.

A chance difference in mortality between two groups of patients

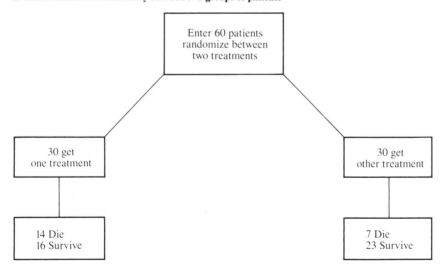

In a report to the Medical Research Council (Britain), it was noted that results at least as extreme as these occur in about 10 per cent of small clinical trials which compare *equivalent* treatments. Variations of this magnitude can be expected as the result of chance allocation of patients at relatively high risk to one treatment group.

The ability of a planned test to distinguish between the merits of two treatments depends on how many patients suffer a relevant 'event' rather than how many patients are enrolled. A committee of Britain's Medical Research Council has emphasized, for instance, that a study with 100 patients, 50 of whom die, is about as sensitive as a study with 1000 patients, 50 of whom succumb.

The discriminating power of a trial also depends on the magnitude of the difference between treatments. The study of a few dozen patients can, in most cases, detect an unusually effective treatment which prevents two thirds of deaths, but more realistic effects, such as preventing about one third of deaths, requires well over 100 patients if the difference is to be detected.

The essence of performing a successful clinical trial, then, is to enroll a sufficient number of *at-risk* patients. I will postpone a discussion of how this 'sufficient number' may be estimated—particularly when there are multiple, and opposing, end-points of interest—until the chapters on The Stopping Rule and on Inferential Decision. The reasoning must be coupled with that used in making inferences from proportional propositions.

Additional 'active' observations

There are almost always a number of outcomes of interest in a formal study that are quite properly classified as 'active' observations, or practice targets. The opportunity to make preliminary observations about the occurrence of such expected events is an important part of every randomized clinical trial. There is, however, a fundamental difference between the two kinds of de-fined targets. The primary outcome is under critical test, but, if no clearly specified pre-trial predictions have been made about the additional 'active' observations, we can hardly claim that they have been in any great danger of refutation.

It is imperative that the additional observations be made, but it is equally necessary that they be clearly labeled as results of a pilot exercise, for it is the 'range' of these latter targets that is under investigation. Further testing is needed to explore the limits of applicability of the newly formed propor-tional propositions.

Oxygen treatment and survival   The relationship between oxygen treatment and survival was a prominent pre-trial concern of the planners of the national controlled RLF trial, but the question was not framed in numerical terms that could be addressed in a formal way. The deaths of infants assigned to two oxygen treatment regimens were monitored week by week during the first three months of the study to determine if there was a systematic difference that could be made out. These *pilot* observations in-dicated only a small disparity in favor of routine (uncurtailed) oxygen treatment. We can now see, with the wisdom of hindsight, how unfortunate it was that these preliminary observations were not followed by focused studies of the survival question.

Intensive treatment and major handicap   The Australian planners of the alternate-assignments trial of intensive care (p 87) stated that they wished to determine if the innovative techniques of 'unproven benefit might even have detrimental effects.' Here the end points of the trial, death and major handicap, were given equal weight, but neither were primary outcome events in the strict sense required for a severe test. Like survival outcome in the RLF trial, the questions in the Australian pilot experience were not number-specific. Twelve years of study (four years of patient intake and eight years of follow-up) provided only an estimate of the range of differences that would be expected in rigorous tests of the *two* questions.

Unpredicted outcomes

The third kind of target event is the most difficult to deal with. On the one hand, the role of serendipity in investigation must not be dismissed. (The princes, in the fairy story *The Three Princes of Serendip*, were always making discoveries, by accidents and sagacity, of things they were not in quest of.) The opportunity to 'dredge' the hard-to-obtain data made available in a well-conducted large clinical trial simply must not be missed. Most commonly, this takes the form of searching for unpredicted associations in many subclasses of enrolled patients. And yet, as probability theorists never tire of warning, we must keep in mind the Fallacy of the Enumeration of Favorable Circumstances—if enough independent phenomena are studied and correlations sought, some will, of course, be found. At the time of an unexpected 'win', it would be well to remember the human drama that takes place in the gambling casino at Monte Carlo. When a patron rakes in a huge pile of chips after an *en plein* bet at the roulette table (thirty five times the amount placed on a single number), a tremble of excitement passes around the room. The 'house' merely yawns, and says, in effect, keep playing.

8 Avoiding entrapment

Decision theory strategists look upon problems in the biological sciences as 'games against nature', and they plan tactics to outwit this capricious adversary. Prudent clinical investigators adopt a similar outlook; they assume that the 'opponent' has planted innocent looking 'traps' to foil planned efforts to separate effects in a comparative study. The suspicious attitude is justified; as I will emphasize by a few more examples, circumstances that mislead in medicine lie in wait to entrap the unwary.

An example of confoundment

In an observation of an effect of detergent on the health of a dog

A woman asked her veterinarian whether it would be safe to wash her dog with a particular detergent. He advised against it, saying it would make the dog sick.

That evening the woman called to say that the dog was ill and asked the vet to come. The woman admitted that, against advice, she had washed the animal with the detergent. The vet shook his head and said, 'I knew it would harm the dog.' 'Oh, I don't think it was the detergent,' said the woman, 'it was putting him in the spin dryer afterward.'
(Related by Edmond A. Murphy of Johns Hopkins University)

TIME-RELATED TRAPS

Intervals before and after start of treatment

Pitfalls related to the element of time are encountered often in studies of the effect of treatments on the duration of life. Here, two segments of time need to be taken into account: the first interval begins with the onset of illness and runs to the beginning of treatment, the second marks the time from initiation of treatment to death. We may be badly misled if we direct our attention solely to a change in the latter period, and fail to consider the marked influence of the timing and efficiency of diagnostic procedures on the elapse of time before treatment. It is not difficult to envisage a change in proportions of the two intervals with no change in the total duration of time from illness onset to death. Age of illness is sometimes more important than chronological age of patients when comparing like with like in clinical trials.

Consider, for example, the results of treatment with an ineffective anti-cancer agent. When a diagnosis of cancer is made early and the useless treatment begins soon after the onset of illness, the drug will appear to prolong life simply because the interval from the start of treatment to death has been made to *seem* relatively long.

Age on enrollment and mortality

Temporal effects are also seen in studies of treatments in newborn infants. Relatively small differences in age on enrollment are associated with exaggerated changes in duration of life. Most deaths occur soon after birth; thus, the probability of survival rises sharply with each passing hour after delivery. When an infant is transferred from the hospital of birth to a special care facility, age on admission may provide a reliable clue to a forecast of the length of life.

Crude versus 'adjusted' mortality rate   A spurious improvement once observed in survival rates of very small babies (under 1.0 kilogram) reared in a large referral center is a case in point. In 1950, only 18 per cent (9/50) of these infants survived in the hospital; two years later the rate rose to 38 per cent (20/53). The improvement was encouraging, and there was much speculation about the cause. However, when corrections were made for the distorting effects of differences in age on admission, the explanation was revealed. The apparent improvement was accounted for by the admission of older, relatively robust infants in the second period of comparison. In fact, the 'adjusted' rates indicated that the survival experience of *comparable* babies was 6 per cent lower in the latter year. (The statistical methods used in the calculation of so-called standardized event-rates—adjusted for age, sex, and so forth—are described in epidemiology textbooks.)

In the same hospital experience, the survival of relatively large infants (1.0–1.5 kilograms) remained unchanged over the period of time under scrutiny (59/81 versus 71/97, 73 per cent survival rate for both years). A comparison of the 'adjusted' rates, however, indicated that there had been a 30 per cent improvement among comparable babies, a finding that was hidden by the discrepancies of age on admission.

Duration of observation

One of the most common 'traps' in medical studies can be found in the details of duration of observation. Most pathological processes take some time to evolve, and patients must remain under observation for a specified period if the manifestation of an abnormal state is to be recognized. When patients are discharged from observation too soon or fail to return at appointed times, the irregularities play havoc with efforts to interpret the frequency of medical events. The distorting effect can be quite subtle.

Incidence of strawberry marks   A trivial but instructive illustration of this kind of entrapment took place in connection with observations made on strawberry marks of the skin (capillary hemangiomas) during the RLF epidemic and immediately thereafter (when occurrence of the eye disorder fell sharply in 1954–5). These minor skin conditions are seen frequently in young infants. They usually appear some days and weeks after birth, grow for a time, and usually disappear spontaneously by the age of two or three years. The 'mark' consists of a tangle of newly-formed blood vessels; under the microscope the appearance is very similar to the exuberant growth of blood vessels in the early stages of RLF. Strawberry hemangiomas seemed to occur more frequently in premature than in full-term babies, and in the late 1940s it was suggested that RLF was nothing more or less than a postnatally-appearing hemangioma of the retina.

In an effort to examine this suggestion systematically, a large special care center began to keep a record of the time of appearance of the superficial marks and to correlate the skin findings with those noted in the eyes of premature infants. The associations were not particularly striking, nonetheless the joint observations were continued over a period of several years. When the occurrence of RLF fell dramatically in late 1954 and in 1955, it was found that the frequency of strawberry marks also declined sharply. These intriguing observations were collated and a draft was made of a report to announce the curious association in a medical journal. As the manuscript was readied for publication, an article was published revealing a 'trap' that had been overlooked.

The new report provided the results of a series of observations made in Sweden on the frequency and time of appearance of skin hemangiomas among 640 prematurely born infants and a control group of 186 mature infants. It was found that weekly examinations for several months after birth in *both* groups revealed no difference in the frequency of occurrence among the premature infants and full size babies. The previously held belief that skin marks were more common in the small infants seemed to be related to length of observation in hospitals. Small babies remained in the hospital for relatively long periods of time after birth and the marks came to medical attention regularly. The large infants left the hospital before the hemangiomas appeared, and frequency among the latter babies was less obvious because they were not assembled in one location.

On the basis of the new insight, the hospital discharge ages of premature infants in the long series about to be reported was examined: the median age at discharge dropped abruptly when the occurrence of RLF fell since infants were no longer kept in the hospital for additional days and weeks to monitor the progress of abnormal eye changes. The report of the 'interesting' change in frequency of skin hemangiomas with restriction of oxygen administration was quietly shelved.

INEQUALITIES IN COMPARED GROUPS

Unequal prognoses

I have noted the strategy of prognostic stratification (p 50) used to sort patients according to susceptibility of suffering an outcome event. Here I wish to emphasize the potential for confusion when unequal groups are compared by relating a hypothetical example given by Feinstein.

Co-mingling patients with unequal prognoses

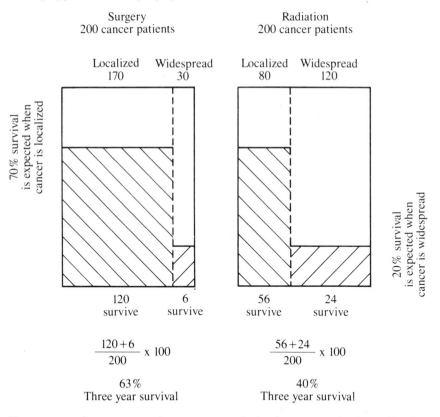

The outcomes of two treatments (surgery versus radiation for cancer, say), when neither has any effect on the natural course of disease, are biased, Feinstein points out, in favor of treatment used in a group of patients in which there is a disproportionate number with relatively good outlook.

Surgery versus radiation for cancer   Suppose, Feinstein argues, the expected
three-year survival rate for patients with a particular cancer is quite high in
those with a growth localized to one site in the body and that the rate is
sharply reduced when the malignant process has spread widely to many
sites. In a comparison of surgical versus radiation treatment, we would
immediately recognize a problem in interpreting the results if surgical treatment was used exclusively for those with localized cancer and radiation was
administered to those with widespread involvement. However, the garbled
effect is not immediately obvious when both kinds of patients are represented in the two treatment groups. The bias will be felt unless the 'mixture'
is proportionately equal in the subgroups with unequal prognostic expectations. A mistaken conclusion about the effectiveness of surgery may come
about solely as a result of our failure to recognize prognostic differences
and disproportionate co-mingling of patients.

Unequal compliance with treatment

The same kind of distortion occurs, Feinstein points out, when there is
unequal compliance with treatments of equal effectiveness in a planned
trial. Suppose, for instance, that success under treatment occurs in many
patients when either A or B maneuver is faithfully maintained and some
improve when treatment is abandoned. If B has such an unappealing taste,
appearance, schedule of administration, and the like, so that it is maintained
by only half of the patients assigned to this regimen, the poor showing of
this group of patients may be attributed, mistakenly, to an inferiority of the
pharmacologic action of the drug.

The adage, there's many a slip 'twixt the cup and the lip (which dates to
the Greek legend of the Argonauts in search of the Golden Fleece) is
applicable here. The issue of compliance is a formidable problem in medical
trials. If it cannot be documented that patients did, in fact, take the drugs
prescribed for them, it would be wise to use some variation of this cautious
wording (and emphasis) in a heading that describes a comparison trial: 'The
outcomes after *prescription* of drugs A and B.'

The combined effects of differences in duration of observation and in
compliance with prescribed treatments have also been described by Feinstein. He warns of compound distortions that may result when precautions
are not taken to avoid potential sources of confoundment.

PRECAUTIONS IN CLINICAL TRIALS

Early in the experience with clinical trials Mainland gave up trying to
catalogue the numerous difficulties that may come up. Instead, he proposed
a list of precautions that might reduce procedural errors (p 68) that occur
so commonly. The guidelines included these categories: choice of investi-

Unequal compliance with prescribed treatments

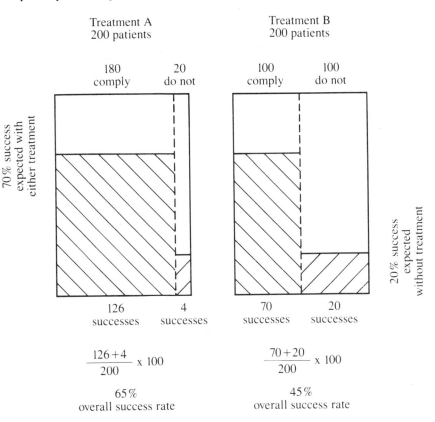

A hypothetical example given by Feinstein of distortion of results caused by differences in patient compliance with prescribed treatments in a trial of two treatments of equal effectiveness.

gators, time for planning, realism in planning, carrying out the plan, and policing the trial.

Although more than twenty years have gone by since he proposed these safeguards, his advice remains timely. The need to improve external relevance requires the involvement of many doctors and more than one hospital in clinical studies—the very situation in which Mainland found that problems multiplied.

Choice of investigators

The personal characteristics of physician investigators, such as motivation, commitment, and acceptance of regimentation are not easily bared, but they are pertinent in large scale trials. The projects cannot be carried out successfully unless the doctors involved are willing to 'freeze' their activities into prescribed molds for a fairly substantial period of time. During this period they are almost certain to be buffeted by stormy forces. Patients, relatives and friends of patients, other physicians, and well-wishers may exert pressure to change treatment when results of other studies become available or when preliminary findings and hopeful leads are widely publicized.

The difficulties are considerable and physicians who are to become involved should have an opportunity to discuss these matters before they agree to participate. The enrolled patients are entitled to an unwavering commitment on the part of their caretakers to carry out a clinical trial faithfully in order to produce interpretable results. Doctors should bow out if there is any question about fulfilling these obligations wholeheartedly.

Additionally, those in charge of a large-scale trial must recruit the support of referring physicians to reduce sampling distortions that may occur over time. As I will discuss later, the active involvement of the medical community is essential if the results are to have an impact on everyday practice at the conclusion of a trial.

Unfortunately, I can do little more than sound these ominous warnings about physician related problems that are a potential source of entrapment in bedside studies. Although there is no ready solution, the difficulties cannot be ignored; it is usually necessary to review the issues periodically during the course of study.

The planning period

A considerable amount of time is needed to plan a medical trial. In one multicenter cancer treatment trial, for instance, one year was allowed for drawing up the protocol (the document containing the agreed upon plan) and the corresponding record-gathering documents. During the year, the planners (physicians and statisticians) met together for one eight-hour day each month. For every hour spent in formal meeting, the planners spent several more in preparation for the working sessions. This pace may seem leisurely and the attention to detail pedantic in the face of the everyday problems of sick and dying patients who cannot wait for an idealized plan, but the worldly pressures simply must be resisted during the hatching period.

Realism in planning

On the other hand, the real world should not be shut out when projecting the proposed conduct of a bedside exercise. The opinions and the behavior of nurses, laboratory technicians, and other health care workers need to be taken into account since their cooperation is indispensable. It is unrealistic to expect that a trial can be carried out without a hitch unless there is fairly complete understanding of the rationale and approval of the goals of an experiment involving a team of caretakers who have a strong sense of duty to protect the welfare of their patients.

Resistance of caretakers A poignant illustration of the need for understanding and cooperation took place in 1952 when the first effort was made to examine the effect of oxygen restriction on RLF occurrence by means of a formal controlled trial. The study was conducted in a large municipal hospital in Washington, D.C. The hospital nursery was staffed by experienced nurses who had been using oxygen liberally in the supportive care of small babies for many years, and they were convinced of the importance of this form of preventive treatment.

When two young investigators carried out the controlled study they discovered, belatedly, that the plan had been contaminated. The nurses believed that the doctors were going to jeopardize the lives of babies assigned to the 'curtailed oxygen' group. At night, some of the older nurses turned the oxygen valves on for babies who were not receiving the gas, then stopped the flow when they went off duty in the morning. Well-meaning resistance of this kind (the word 'sabotage' is unfair) is not at all rare, and it may go undetected if a trial is not closely monitored.

Practical limit At an early stage in the step by step development of information about two treatments, reality often imposes a practical limit on the specificity of the question addressed in a comparative trial. For example, Peto and co-workers noted that a realistic question may be, Is it better to adopt a *policy* of Treatment A if possible, with deviations if necessary, or a *policy* of Treatment B if possible, with deviations if necessary, for patients who seem to have a particular disorder?

This wobbly question concerning management may be more relevant for the moment than a higher order question, Is A better than B for the disorder? The refined question must simply wait until physicians and patients are ready to follow narrowly prescribed policies in future trials.

Irregularities in the trial plan

In a pragmatic trial, an accounting should be made of all patients who are considered for enrollment, including those who do not satisfy the requirements for prescribed treatments. I mentioned the problem of 'irregulars' earlier, now I wish to distinguish between exclusions, withdrawals, and losses.

Exclusions Patients excluded before randomization do not bias the treatment comparison. However, it is important to report the number of patients

Exclusions, withdrawals, and losses

In a pragmatic (management policy) trial

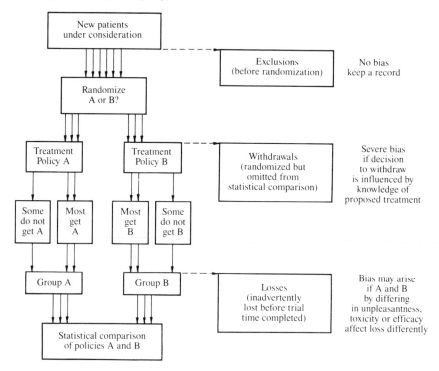

(Redrawn from Peto and co-workers' report to Britain's Medical Research Council)

left out and the reasons given for exclusion in order to make comparisons with other series.

Withdrawals Patients deliberately removed from a trial after randomization cannot be dismissed from consideration easily. Results may be distorted by the absence of such post-allotment withdrawals. It is necessary, for instance, to adopt an explicit rule to deal with conditions which are difficult to diagnose. If a review indicates that a patient was enrolled on the basis of an error in diagnosis, the participant may be withdrawn and classified as an 'exclusion'. However, we need to be assured that this decision was not influenced by knowledge of the treatment that the patient would have received.

The working rules about all withdrawals (especially partially treated patients who defect) need to be carefully thought out and specified in some detail to guard against systematic bias. .

Losses Patients who do not return for specified follow-up examination present an awkward problem in medical studies. Although it is the common practice, for instance, to accept the length of life prior to loss in a comparison (using a life-table correction for duration of observation), this is not completely satisfactory because the lost patients may turn out to be a special class. No effort should be spared to document the fate of patients who disappear. The considerable time and expense needed to pursue missing patients should be regarded as essential investments.

Conventions concerning deviations

In discussing procedural biases, I noted that it is unrealistic to expect error-free treatments in a planned trial and I presented the argument that in a pragmatic trial the results of the treated-by-error patients should be included in the results for assigned treatment, despite the mistake. Disagreement about this point is common, but the logic is fairly straightforward. Peto pointed out that, when all the deviants are retained, the conclusions will be changed only if deviations are more numerous in one treatment group than in another and if the outcome in the deviants differs markedly from that in protocol-adherents. But in both of these circumstances, disclaiming the deviants is certainly not justifiable. Thus, removal of protocol-deviants becomes either irrelevant or invalid, and the safe general rule is to retain the results of all randomized patients in the final numerical analysis.

It is often of interest to describe the results among those who received treatments exactly as prescribed. But this is a data-dredging operation; there is no valid way in which the laws of probability may be invoked to help with the interpretation of any differences found in such a selected comparison.

Standard criteria for deviations I should point out that efforts must be made to regularize departures from described treatments whenever possible. For instance, an 'index of failure' of treatment may be devised and adopted as a practical end point. The convention avoids the confusion introduced by auxilliary treatments given when death is thought to be imminent. When the criteria for treatment 'failure' have been satisfied, the patient has completed his or her trial time; treatments and outcomes beyond this point are described, but they are not reckoned in formal results.

Unfortunately, this is only a partial solution to the problem of irregularity. If we are unable to guard against unequal application of the 'failure' criteria, the results may become hopelessly tangled.

Policing the trial

Mainland emphasized the need for a highly visible overseer to reduce the risk of unexpected entrapment in the conduct of treatment trials. The on-site coordinator may be given various titles, but his duties should be those of a policeman: to prevent trouble, to catch it quickly when it starts, and to be always ready to give immediate help when it is needed. Moreover, he must snoop into every detail of the on-going trial as he 'walks his beat'.

Randomized clinical trials are exceptionally difficult to carry out because they require restrained behavior on the part of a profession that is licensed by society to act in an unrestrained manner to relieve human suffering. The duties of 'law enforcement' are sometimes assigned to a statistician, but I suggest that this is quite unfair. The 'night stick' belongs in the hand of a physician who is thoroughly familiar with all of the details of the current study and the deliberations that led to the wording of the protocol. And, most importantly, he must have an intimate knowledge about the setting in which the studies are carried out, including good insight into the character of each of the doctors, nurses, and others involved in the project, if he is to be effective in the prevention of systematic errors.

Coordination center In a multicenter trial, an executive unit must be designated to coordinate the exercise. This coordination center, which is usually physically separate from the participating institutions, receives, processes, edits, and analyzes data generated in the trial; and it provides epidemiological, statistical, and computational guidance. A central laboratory may be required to insure uniform observations of defined criteria (these may include chemical analyses, coding of x-rays and electrocardiograms, and so forth). A large-scale trial also requires a committee of experts, a detailed

---

Clinical trial committee
Specialist members in a complex multicenter trial

Expert clinician for field surveillance
Clinical pharmacologist
Epidemiologist
Biostatistician
Pathologist
End point specialist (e.g. electrocardiography . . .)
Laboratory specialist
Computer specialist
Expert in classification of disease
Medicolegal expert
Ethicist
Patient representative
(From Christian R. Klimt, University of Maryland)

organizational structure (such as a policy board, steering committee, data and safety monitoring committee, and quality control group), and a clearly defined chain of command to control the multifold activities of the complex operation. Patients who agree to participate in a planned experiment deserve the assurance that 'law and order' are policed on their behalf.

9 The stopping rule

It would be reckless to set the ponderous machinery of a randomized clinical trial into motion without some thought about how it is to be halted. The dilemma faced by doctors has a familiar form. If a treatment trial is stopped too soon, the harmful consequences or hoped-for benefits of the innovation will be overlooked; if it is too prolonged, patients who continue to receive the old treatment are denied the new benefits, or unnecessary numbers of patients are exposed to the inferior new agent under test.

And Elijah came unto all the people, and said,
How long halt ye between two opinions? If the Lord *be* God follow him: but if Baal, *then* follow him. And the people answered him not a word.

I *Kings* 18:21

What is needed is some sort of a stopping rule that will limit the magnitudes of these opposing risks; it is completely unrealistic to expect that we can step into the unknown with perfect safety. And the rule must be devised with what may seem like imperious vacuity reminiscent of the King of Hearts' directive to the White Rabbit in *Alice in Wonderland*: 'Begin at the beginning,' the King said, gravely, 'and go on till you come to the end, then stop.'

There are, in fact, two situations for which plans must be formulated: the stopping point of a pilot trial and the termination point in a fully mounted formal trial. The first circumstance is often neglected because the relatively formless first steps of innovation are not perceived as requiring a pre-planned limit.

SIZE OF A PILOT TRIAL

The prime objective of a preliminary exercise is to rehearse a proposed trial in order to uncover unforeseen difficulties that may arise. But there is additional information that needs to be rooted out in a pilot experience: we must have some rough estimate of the size of difference in outcomes that is to be expected under the treatments on trial. This estimate provides the reasonable basis for settling on a number-specific question which will be tested.

Setting a limit in advance

Obviously, it is impossible to make a *calculation* beforehand of the amount of experience required to hone the operations and provide a realistic esti-mate of the expected difference. It is necessary, nevertheless, to make a firm declaration about the dimensions of a pilot trial before it is launched. The information available from past experience and from pre-clinical tests in animals may be used to help with the judgment for setting a limit.

The exploratory phase, I said earlier, should not be open-ended because it is too easily misguided. When a run of favorable outcomes occurs under a novel treatment, there is an understandable temptation to continue and include the results of the pilot trial in the legitimate rolls of the full exercise. When the first outcomes after an innovation seem no better or are worse than the standard approach, there is strong pressure to abandon the follow-through plan for an authentic test. These attitudes act as stumbling blocks to an ordered progression of evaluation; and the obstacles are en-countered particularly often when the exploration of a new treatment is conducted without concurrent controls.

> You can prove almost anything with the evidence of a small enough segment of time. How often in the search for truth, the answer of the minute is positive, the answer of the hour qualified, the answers of the year contradictory!
>
> Edwin Way Teale

A 'dramatic breakthrough' A snowball effect of early success was seen when a new treatment to support the oxygenation of newborn infants with severe respiratory distress was introduced in 1969. Slight continuous posi-tive pressure was applied to the airway of infants with the condition called 'hyaline membrane disease' to counter the pathologic forces in this disorder that tend to collapse the lung during the exhalatory phase of each cycle of respiration. Only about one quarter of infants with severe symptoms were expected to recover. The first infant treated in this way survived; in 1970, the results of treating seven babies (six of whom recovered) were reported to the medical community; and in 1971, the results of treating 20 babies (16 of whom lived) were published in full.

This new approach was adopted by physicians quickly and widely; testi-monial reports of favorable experiences appeared in medical journals throughout the world. Five years later a reviewer concluded that the weight of confirmatory evidence (based on historical comparisons) seemed over-whelming, and this form of treatment was declared a major breakthrough in the care of distressed infants. The claims, however, were not supported by the results found in the few controlled clinical trials that were later conducted to evaluate the limits of applicability of the positive-pressure technique. The advantage over conventional methods of ventilatory support was quite modest.

The problem in conditions with high mortality

When new treatment for a highly fatal condition shows promising results in a pilot trial, an argument is often made against stopping to carry out the formalities of a randomized trial. (Such an 'unjustified-risk' argument was made after the encouraging early results of positive-pressure treatment were made known in 1970 and 1971.) There is nothing particularly illogical about this reasoning if we can accept the premises on which the argument is based. However, as we have seen, wholly regular events in medicine are quite rare. Moreover, the classification of clinical states are subject to con-siderable leeway in interpretation. Unlike the situation in meningeal tuber-culosis before streptomycin (p 44), the definition of an 'invariably fatal condition' is often imprecise and the label is applied loosely. Uncertainty in diagnosis, particularly early in the course of illness, is common.

Recognition of mild cases   A Boston group observed that patients with severe and fatal disease merely represent the 'tip of an iceberg'. There are almost always many more with milder forms of the same disease, and increased interest in diagnosis takes place when a new treatment is intro-duced. This invariably leads to the recognition of less severely involved patients who were previously overlooked (most of the unheralded patients recovered spontaneously). Consequently, outcome in currently treated per-sons appears improved as compared with previous experience, even when treatment is without effect or is actually deleterious.

With hindsight, a strong case could have been made for the use of a randomized control design from the very outset of the pilot trial of positive-pressure treatment. The conservative approach would have pro-vided a hedge against unknown risks, and the concurrent control design would have guarded against the possibility that a progressive shift in sever-ity of disease among the twenty babies enrolled over the sixteen-month period of the initial observations might distort the estimate of expected difference in outcome.

Preparation for a strong challenge

On the working assumption that there are no universally applicable, perfect treatments, the goal of critical experimentation is to flush out weakness and

An idealized model of medical diagnosis

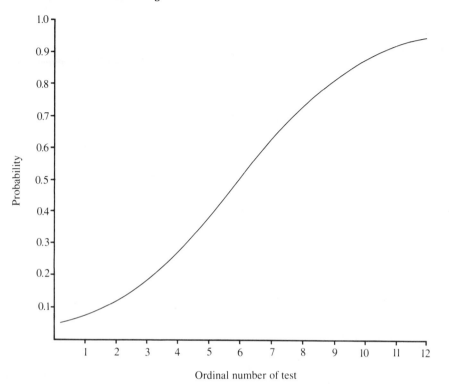

Ordinal number of test

Given certain evidence from a patient with a single disease, a doctor formulates questions and carries out a number of tests. Evidence in favor of the disease may thus be elicited at a constant rate: the probability of the presence of the disease then increases as a symmetrical S-shaped curve. W.I. Card and I.J. Good of the University of Glasgow point out that it is not known on which part of the curve a doctor usually works when he makes a diagnosis.

limits in new proposals. We have seen that it is difficult to mount a strong challenge when the question posed by an innovation is posed in general form. The numberless question, Does the new technique of positive-pressure improve the survival of distressed babies? is relatively safe from the risk of refutation until it is recast in quantitative terms.

Patients who first receive the untried treatment are asked to act as an advance party to scout the general question and bring back information for use in formulating a specific version that has an increased probability of exposing limitations. There may need to be several forays to generate information about the details of treatment (such as timing and dosage) before a vulnerable question is framed: Does the new technique, administered in the manner specified, improve survival from about 25 per cent to approximately 80 per cent?

This process of angling for a model based on observations of events as they occur is similar to the hypothesis-seeking 'fishing expedition' (p 20) using events that occurred some time in the past, and the same precautions about interpretation apply. Any preliminary search of observations makes it difficult to evaluate results of statistical tests on the same collection of information.

SIZE OF A RANDOMIZED CLINICAL TRIAL

The focus of interest in estimating the proper size of clinical experiments is not quite the same as that in the formal procedure used by statisticians for determining how many observations are required to decide whether or not to reject a hypothesis. Zelen has pointed out that many so-called hypothesis-testing situations in the world of medical events are in reality 'estimation of difference' problems.

Null hypothesis versus limits of difference

In the classic hypothesis testing procedure we start with a general question structured in the form of a disclaimer, called the null hypothesis; for instance, positive-pressure treatment is neither more nor less effective than standard management. Then we specify the conditions for deciding whether or not to reject this assertion as true. In a pragmatic trial we are not primarily interested in the truth of hypotheses. When two methods of management are compared, we want to know the limits of their difference, for it is extremely unlikely that they will bring about effects that are *exactly equal*.

We are forced to concede, therefore, that in clinical matters the null hypothesis is rarely, if ever, true. In the example of the positive-pressure treatment, there was every reason to expect, from the outset, that it would not give results that were exactly the same as standard management. The goal of a formal test is to provide an estimate of some magnitude of difference that will have practical importance in general application. This target is within reach of the randomized clinical trial. The weightier questions concerning the status of hypotheses are simply left hanging—it is impractical to test them exhaustively at the bedside.

Despite this caveat, it is useful to *begin* the design of an experiment from the hypothesis-testing point of view. The reasoning used in the theoretical model allows us to make a preliminary calculation of the size of a clinical trial. The first approximation of dimensions serves as a solid point of departure for some thought about the medical and community implications of results of the proposed project. The final size, which emerges after completion of fairly wide-ranging consultations, is likely to give rise to a stopping rule that is unique for each clinical trial.

Rough estimate of the number of patients to enroll in a controlled trial

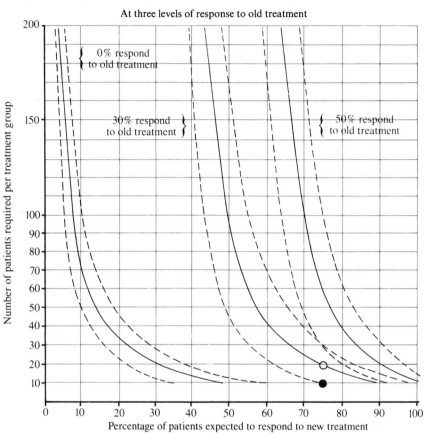

At three levels of response to old treatment

The vertical scale indicates the number of patients required in *each* treatment group, and the horizontal scale notes the proportion of patients expected to respond to the new treatment. The three sets of curves depict situations in which the proportions of responses to old treatment are 0, 30, and 50 per cent.

In each set, the solid line curve indicates the relationships when the chances* for detecting the specified differences are 4 out of 5, the dashed line to the left when the chances for successful detection are only 1 out of 2, and the dashed line to the right in each set when the chances for a decisive result are 95 out of 100.

For example (○), when 30 per cent of babies respond to old management and 75 per cent are expected to recover under the new treatment, if 20 patients are enrolled in each group (that is, a total of 40 patients in the trial), the chances are reasonably good (4 out of 5) that the difference will be detected in a trial of this size. If only 10 patients are enrolled in *each* group (●), the chances are merely 1 out of 2 that a 'statistically significant' result will be obtained. Compiled by C.J. Clark and Colin C. Downie of Imperial Chemical Industries (Britain).

*In these calculations the risk level for Type I error is set at 5 per cent. Levels for Type II error are: solid line 20 per cent (power 0.8), dashed line to the left 50 per cent (power 0.5), and dashed line to the right 5 per cent (power 0.95). There is agreement that a two-sided test of 'significance' will be performed on the results (that is, we wish to detect differences in both directions, improvement or worsening with the new treatment).

Smallest number of patients to enroll in a controlled clinical trial

At specified responses to each of two treatments

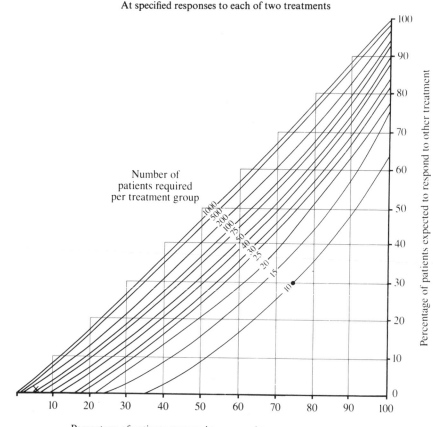

Number of
patients required
per treatment group

Percentage of patients expected to respond to other treatment

Percentage of patients expected to respond to one treatment

The vertical and horizontal scales indicate the contrasting proportions of patients expected to respond to two compared treatments. The number of patients required in *each* treatment group for a 1 out of 2 chance* of detecting the specified difference is indicated by the set of curves. The greater of two percentage responses is always plotted against the horizontal scale when using this graph.

For example (●), when a 30 per cent versus 75 per cent response contrast is expected under two treatments, 10 patients in *each* group would be needed for 1 out of 2 chances of obtaining a 'statistically significant'* result. On the other hand (X), when a 1 per cent versus 5 per cent treatment response contrast is expected, more than 100 patients in *each* group are needed at the same risk levels.

Compiled by Clark and Downie.

* In these calculations the risk level for Type I error is set at 5 per cent. The level for Type II error is 50 per cent (relatively low power 0.5); and a two-sided test of significance will be carried out on results.

Idealized calculation of trial size

In the idealized approach we are obliged, before the trial begins, to provide arbitrary answers to three questions that will come up at the end of the exercise. First, if we say at the end of a trial, 'There is an important difference in outcomes,' how large a risk of being wrong are we willing to take? In the event the declaration is mistaken, we have committed a Type I error; the probability of this risk is reported as α, the 'significance level' adopted in the trial.

Second, how large a risk are we willing to take in missing the actual existence of an important difference by declaring 'No statistically significant difference'? A mistake of this kind is called a Type II error; the probability of the second risk is termed β.

Finally, before the trial commences, we must answer the question, What is the smallest difference we regard as important enough to find? The difference between outcome under standard treatment and the new treatment is designated as Δ.

The answers to the three questions provide the information required for a laborious calculation of trial size. Statistical texts summarize the results of the arithmetic in the form of sample-size-needed tables; these indicate the *minimal* number of patients to enroll in a clinical trial at various risk levels adopted for the two types of error and the specified difference in treatment outcomes.

Chances of detecting a specified difference The term 'power of the test' $(1 - \beta)$ appears in sample size tables and graphs to indicate the probability of detecting a specified difference. Stated another way 'power' expresses the chances of avoiding a Type II error. When we adopt a relatively low risk level for β (say 0.05), the detecting 'power' of the trial is quite high $(1 - 0.05 = 0.95)$. The sample-size-needed calculations make it clear that improved chances of uncovering the true difference in a clinical trial can only be achieved by increasing the number of patients enrolled.

Trial size and 'negative' results Jennie A. Freiman and collaborators at Mount Sinai School of Medicine reviewed 71 'negative' randomized clinical trials; the observed differences between the proposed and the control treatments were not large enough to satisfy a specified 'significance' level (the risk of a Type I error) and the results were declared to be 'not statistically significant'. Analysis of these clinical studies indicated that the investigators often worked with numbers of enrolled patients too small to offer a reasonable chance of avoiding the opposing mistake, a Type II error. Fifty of the trials had a greater than 10 per cent risk of missing a substantial difference (true discrepancy of 50 per cent) in treatment outcome. The reviewers warned that many treatments labeled as 'no different from control' have not received a critical test because the trials used had insufficient 'power' to do the job intended.

PRACTICAL ASPECTS OF TRIAL SIZE ESTIMATION

When the limits imposed by the inexorable laws of probability have been determined (from the results of the statistical arithmetic displayed in sample-size-needed tables), we must turn to face the realities imposed by the everyday world. And these mundane considerations must extend to the long-term perspective of the community at large: its goals and its resources.

Magnitude of an 'important' difference

What does the statement 'clinically important difference' mean? Obviously, the notion of what we will consider 'important' is as difficult to capture as a greased pig. Unfortunately, we cannot circumvent the slippery task, for the magnitude of the 'important' difference is often the most crucial issue in planning and evaluating the clinical trial.

A Procrustean approach is often used to define the size of an 'important' difference by an inverted process. Doctors begin by estimating the limit of trial size (for example, the number of patients available in one institution over the period of time they can devote to the study) and from this number they determine the smallest difference that can be detected at various risk levels for the two types of error. This ad hoc approach to the definition of an 'important' difference should be avoided because it tends to promote trials with low 'power'. Whenever possible, multicenter trials should be carried out to overcome restrictions on numbers of patients available.

The size of difference in outcome specified in an upcoming trial should reflect a view of public gain or loss. In every case we must consider that when a medical experiment is completed and the report is published, it ceases to be an isolated decision problem. It has been said that the experimenter pays the piper and calls the tune he likes best; but the music is broadcast so that others may listen. Thus, we must ask, How much of its resources is the community willing to invest to achieve a specified improvement in outcome?

The question is not foreign to community planners who must advise about investments whenever an intervention is proposed to improve the outlook for citizens. The reasoning is the same when the issue is a new project to reduce automobile accident-related deaths and disabilities or a new treatment to reduce untoward outcomes related to premature birth.

Qualitative aspects of 'importance'

A clear distinction between pragmatic and explanatory emphasis is not always possible in a clinical trial. Under such ambiguous conditions, the definition of an 'important' difference requires some review from the point of view of the underlying theories about the pathologic process that is under study. For example, in evaluating the effect of treatment on RLF, which of two outcome indicators will provide more important practical as well as explanatory information: the frequently occurring early blood vessel changes, which often subside, or the less frequent manifestation of scarring, which is irreversible?

In order to detect a specified reduction in occurrence of RLF, we will need relatively few patients if we choose vascular changes as the indicator; many more patients must be enrolled to detect a difference in scarring, the more rarely occurring end point. But the two indicators provide different kinds of information about the disorder because the relationship between the early changes and scarring is not a simple one (for example, there is good reason to suspect that the agent which initiates the blood vessel abnormalities is unable to produce the scarring complications in the absence of an additional operative factor).

I suggest that only such far-ranging considerations by community pragmatists and by medical theorists provide a practical solution to the difficult problem of fixing the value of the 'important' difference in a randomized clinical trial.

From these remarks it will be obvious that the arbitrary values chosen for the probabilities of committing Type I and Type II errors are subject to the same review: risk levels in the formula used to calculate trial size must take into account the implications for community well-being and for medical theory. Again, the risk levels chosen exert a sharp effect on the estimate.

Multiple end points

Before leaving the considerations involved in fashioning a stopping rule, I must call attention to the fact that I have confined the arguments to a single end point of interest. A number of difficulties are introduced by multiple end points in a clinical trial. In addition to the issue of whether or not pre-trial predictions were made, there are complications that relate to the matter of a stopping rule.

Trial size in conflicting outcomes   At a time when the frequency of RLF in the United States was relatively high (before 1955), a small randomized clinical trial was conducted in a single hospital to test the effect of oxygen management policy in reducing the risk of eye damage. The results sup-

High *versus* low oxygen

RLF and Survival

	Oxygen management	
	High	Low
No. enrolled	45	40
Survived	36 (80%)	28 (70%)
RLF	8 (22%)	0 (0)

A small randomized clinical trial was conducted in a single hospital in 1953–4. Babies in 'high oxygen' received this treatment for two weeks after birth; 'low oxygen' was given only for cyanosis (blue discoloration of the skin). It was concluded that the difference in survival rates in the two groups was 'not statistically significant'.

8 of 36 surviving infants (22 per cent) developed scarring RLF after 'high oxygen' treatment; there were no instances of the disorder among 28 babies in the 'low oxygen' group.

It could be said before this trial began, the chances of detecting a reduction in occurrence of RLF from 22 per cent to 0 are about 95 out of 100 with about 40 babies in each oxygen management group. However, for merely 1 out of 2 chances of detecting a 'statistically significant' difference in survival from 80 per cent to 70 per cent, well over 100 infants in each group will be required (risk level for Type I error set at 5 per cent, for Type II error at 50% = power 0.5).

ported the prediction that this risk would be reduced by a policy of oxygen restriction. Far too few infants, however, were enrolled to evaluate an adverse effect of the new policy on survival.

We can envision the mirror image of this disturbing problem of trial size in conflicting outcomes, at a time when the frequency of RLF was quite low, as indeed it was when positive pressure treatment was introduced in 1969. If this new treatment that improved the oxygenation of premature infants had been evaluated in a controlled trial, both survival *and RLF* would have been important end points of immediate interest. Here, the smallest number required for even odds of detecting an increase in survival from, say, 30 per cent to 75 per cent would be 10 infants in each group. But the number needed to detect the possibility of a five-fold increase in RLF blindness in the same babies (say from 1 per cent to 5 per cent) would have been over 100 patients enrolled in each group.

THE MULTIPLE-LOOK DILEMMA

In describing the process of determining trial size, I have made the assumption that the dimensions are rigidly fixed before the project begins. Now we need to examine some of the difficulties that arise with such fixed sample size plans.

The occurrence of temporary trends in favor of one of two compared treatments is guaranteed by the laws of probability, even when equally effective treatments are compared. (In the behavior of perfect coins, runs of 'heads' and 'tails' *must* occur in a series of tosses.) In order to guard against expectancy effects (p 65) that are introduced when physicians and nurses become aware of such trends as a trial progresses, it is literally necessary to hide the accumulating data. This is very difficult to carry out; in many circumstances, conscientious caretakers are well aware of which treatment is 'ahead'. Moreover, only an investigator with superhuman will power can refrain from 'peeking' at the results from time to time in the course of a long clinical trial.

'Peeking'

The director or overseeing group is tempted to analyze the results repeatedly as they accumulate and to stop the trial the moment 'statistical significance' is achieved (before the pre-trial requirements for a fixed sample size have been met). The motives for these actions are irreproachable; the number of patients exposed to an inferior treatment should be kept to a minimum, and patients should be protected from undertaking risks that were unforeseen when the trial was designed. But a penalty must be paid for these well-intentioned monitoring measures, and the price of 'peeking' is often overlooked.

Prevention of sudden death after heart attack   The problem was exemplified by the experience of a large multicenter controlled study of a new drug to prevent sudden death among patients with a recent heart attack (myocardial infarction). The researchers performed interim analyses of the results as they accumulated.

In early 1978, the outcomes appeared to favor the new agent, sulfinpyrazone, and the question of whether or not to continue had to be faced. In the absence of a predetermined stopping rule, the investigators settled their dilemma by submitting the results to a prestigious medical journal. The agony-torn researchers were quoted as saying that if the magazine accepted the findings as 'statistically valid', the experiment would be halted!

Inevitability of 'statistical significance'   When accumulating data are tested repeatedly, 'statistical significance' *will be achieved* if the testing continues indefinitely. This flat statement applies no matter how improbable a 'significance' criterion we choose, and regardless of whether or not there is any difference in the effects of two treatments under test.

In essence, as an analyst provides the goddess of fortune with repeated opportunities for action during the collection of results, the likelihood of

The 'peeking' problem

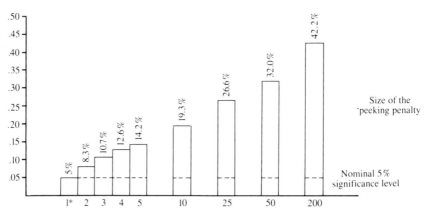

Number of times the accumulating data are analyzed for 'statistical significance'

* Data analyzed once at pre-determined fixed sample-size point

Change in probability (expressed as percentage) of achieving a positive result, wholly by chance, after repeated (serial) testing for 'statistical significance'. The conventional pre-trial risk level of 5 per cent for Type I error is premised on a once-and-for-all significance test. After the tenth 'peek' at accumulating results the nominal 5 per cent greatly underestimates the probability of a chance effect: it is now over 19 per cent. The chances climb to over 42 per cent by the 200th attempt to analyze accumulating data.
Calculated by McPherson.

achieving a positive result wholly by chance increases progressively. The situation is not unlike that in horse racing; all the rules of the race must be agreed to in advance, and all bets made before the starting bell. Bettors who declare that the race is over when their horse is ahead have trouble collecting their money.

Adjustment for specified 'peeks' A way of overcoming the penalty of multiple analyses while retaining the option of stopping a trial early was suggested by Klim McPherson while at the Medical Research Council (Britain): shift the nominal level of 'significance' at which the trial will be stopped. For example, it is decided *in advance of a trial* that a 5 per cent risk level of committing a Type I error will be maintained, and the accumulating data will be examined for 'statistical significance' on five occasions. McPherson calculates that under these conditions, a risk level of a bit more than $1\frac{1}{2}$ per cent will be required in any one of the five tests of 'significance', if the pre-trial Type I error risk level of 5 per cent is to be safeguarded faithfully.

Adjusted 'significance' levels after repeated tests on accumulating results

		Number of repeated 'significance' tests											
	1	2	3	4	5	6	7	8	9	10	15	20	100
Pre-trial level of 'significance' (%)	1	0.56	0.41	0.33	0.28	0.25	0.23	0.21	0.20	0.19	0.15	0.13	0.06
	5	2.96	2.21	1.83	1.59	1.42	1.30	1.20	1.13	1.07	0.86	0.75	0.32
	10	6.01	4.62	3.85	3.37	3.04	2.80	2.60	2.45	2.32	1.88	1.66	0.72

Given the pre-trial 'significance' levels of 1, 5, and 10 per cent (risk levels for Type I error), the adjusted value needed at stated numbers of repeated tests is provided in the body of the table.

By the tenth test on accumulating results, a level of 1.07 per cent must be achieved to maintain a pre-trial risk level of 5 per cent for Type I error.

Calculated by McPherson.

Sequential analysis

Another approach to the multiple-look dilemma in medical experiments is to adopt a stopping rule designed to permit 'continuous peeking' as the trial proceeds. The scheme is based on a section of statistical theory known as sequential analysis, developed largely by Abraham Wald and the Statistical Research Group at Columbia University in the 1940s. The practical problem addressed by the theorists was the sampling procedure used in industry for quality control; sequential procedures of inspection were developed that used the results of drawing articles from an assembly line to decide whether or not sampling should continue.

In sequential plans adapted for clinical trials, sample size is not fixed in advance. The results are inspected continuously and the trial halts according to predetermined rules decided by the choice of risk levels for Type I and Type II errors and specification of a clinically important difference. The method usually leads to economy in testing. On the average, fewer observations are required to reach a decision; but the 'savings', it should be noted, are not certain. The likelihood of reducing the number of patients who must be exposed to poor treatments is an attractive argument in favor of sequential medical trials.

Limitations of monitoring designs

Sequential plans (and the adaptive designs for allotment which I mentioned earlier, p 55) are limited to the kinds of clinical situations in which the outcome of treatment can be assessed fairly soon. If the diagnosis of the result must be delayed, the entire reason for the continuous monitoring strategy is lost (unnecessary enrollments continue while waiting for undecided outcomes).

Critics of sequential medical trials have pointed out that the approach allows only a single target of response in devising a stopping rule. But this drawback applies to all focused experiments. Phased approaches need to be devised to test multiple questions, particularly when conflicting outcomes must be taken into account.

Much of the desperation felt by bedside researchers who are struggling to devise a stopping rule is summed up by the comments of one group involved in a large scale trial; 'Once you terminate this, you're up against it: You can never do it this way again!' The long-term costs of this now-or-never restriction deserve careful analysis.

10   Inferential decision

DECISIVE AMOUNT OF EVIDENCE

I have used quotation marks to set off the word 'significance' and the phrase 'statistically significant' to signal that these terms (referring to an amount of evidence obtained in a test that we will accept as decisive) are easily misinterpreted. The confusion, I believe, stems from our desperate longing for anchors of certainty in a sea of doubt. We hope that if we go to the considerable trouble of conducting a comparative trial and observe the rules of evidence scrupulously, we will arrive at a point where we can stop and come to an unequivocal decision. We dream of moving from doubt to certitude about the questioned events, an action that is epitomized by the declaration, 'We have achieved a significant result.'

Random error and systematic bias

Unfortunately, the telegraphic message conceals more than it reveals about the nature of verdicts made after clinical trials. For example, it may hide the fact that a 'significance' test is not a magical operation to determine whether or not there was some hidden bias in the investigation.

When a statistical test is applied like a recipe in a cook book, without first examining the experimental design used to reduce the influence of extraneous factors, the computation is a futile exercise (p 27). The mechanical practice reflects a commonly held opinion that effects revealed in experimental data are due only to factors under test plus chance (strictly random error). But a decision statement expressed in terms of probability has nothing useful to say about the role of chance unless we can be assured that random effects have not been overwhelmed by extraneous systematic influences.

Terminology   If it were possible to outlaw the word 'significant' when describing statistical inferences, the ban would go a long way in improving the clarity of our assertions about the state of evidence in medicine. (Mainland once proposed that the ambiguous and grandiloquent term 'significance test' be replaced by the more specific and explanatory title of 'random frequency test'.) But the unfortunate word is embedded in thought and in writing; little can be done except to sound warnings about the referents of the value-laden expression. Not the least of the difficulties is the confusion between 'statistical significance' and 'practical significance'; the two are not always congruent.

The 0.05 threshold of 'significance'

An illusory concept is that of a critical threshold of rarity (a 1-in-20 risk of Type I error stated as 'significant at the $\alpha = 0.05$ level'), as opposed to the notion of a gradient of improbability with no discernible 'break' in increasing odds against the likelihood that a specified event has occurred wholly by chance.

The use of verdict terms in statistical analyses of biologic problems was traced by Mainland to a paper written by Karl Pearson in 1896 in which differences in measurements of the human body were stated to be 'significant' or 'not significant' by reference to a quantity called the probable error. A 'significant' difference came to be defined as one that occurred rarely when random samples were taken from the same population, and 'rare' was defined later as outside the range of two standard deviations. This range excludes slightly less than 5 per cent of the total number of sample observations (about $2\frac{1}{2}$ per cent in each outlying 'tail' of the distribution, p 32).

R.A. Fisher adopted the custom and wrote, 'We shall not often be astray if we draw a conventional line at 0.05 and consider that ... [lower] values ... indicate a real discrepancy ... It is convenient to take this [0.05] point as a limit in judging whether a deviation is to be considered significant or not.'

Thus, the choice of the threshold level for Type I error owes more to historical custom than to some inflexible characteristic of data; the cut-off standard, it has been noted, it not a law of Nature. The choice of how often we are willing to 'be astray' is ours, and this determination cannot be made rationally without examining the possible consequences of our decision.

SELECTION OF A 'SIGNIFICANCE' TEST

Before discussing the selection of standards of rarity, I should point out that the choice of the probability-measuring instrument—the 'significance' test—requires some thought. And these deliberations must take place *before* the collection of information begins. The assumptions concerning sampling distribution and sample size that underlie the commonly used tests are described in textbooks of statistics; and these pre-conditions guide the choice of a computational procedure for making statistical inferences.

Badgering the data

Nothing prevents us from performing arithmetic operations on any and all numbers obtained in a series of observations or a formal comparative trial. After the collection of data, we are not physically restrained from shopping for the 'significance' test that turns out the most impressive values when our numbers are plugged into the innocent formulae. But we cannot, in good conscience, lean on the laws of probability for support in the interpretation of such illegally derived results. A wag observed that almost any set of data, if sufficiently badgered, can be exhausted into submission.

Parametric and nonparametric tests

'Parametric significance test' is the term applied to a method that assumes some *particular* distribution of variables. (The word parameter refers to a specific value of a characteristic in a parent population.) The assumption is made that the frequency distribution of variables (height, for instance) in the parent population from which our patients are drawn has a bell-shaped symmetry (confusingly termed a 'normal' distribution). Although parametric tests are accurate in many situations in which characteristics of interest are not symmetrically distributed, the tests are weakened when the population distributions are markedly distorted and when very small sample sizes are analyzed.

Since these limiting conditions are commonly encountered in medical problems, nonparametric tests (which are developed without reference to the distributions of variables) have a distinct advantage. The distributions of age at death and the ordinally ranked grades of RLF are examples of the kinds of asymmetries which turn up frequently in event measurements. The most widely used nonparametric technique is the χ^2 test for categorical data, that is, 'success', 'failure'; another is the Wilcoxon test for ranked ordinal data; these and others are described in statistical texts.

CHOOSING A LEVEL OF 'SIGNIFICANCE'

The choice of a rarity level that will be called 'significant' in a clinical trial involves a thoroughgoing analysis of the actions contemplated by decision makers. In an applied field like medicine, we are obliged to consider the price we are willing to pay if our future actions turn out to be wrong. The gambling analogy is inescapable: prudent bettors examine their bankrolls and decide how much they are prepared to risk before setting the terms of a bet.

Weighing consequences

If the consequence of being wrong about a treatment involves a relatively small loss to future patients and to the community (such as frequent failure to shorten the course of a benign disease that usually subsides spontaneously, minor risk of treatment-induced complications, and small expenditure of personal and community resources), the risk level for Type I error may be set at, say, $P \leq 0.10$ (the capital letter P, for probability level, is the conventional label for the value). We can afford to take the risk of being wrong 10 per cent of the time when we declare that treatments of this kind are effective. As the potential cost of incorrect decisions increases, however, we wish to lower the risk of Type I error accordingly. The customary 5 per cent 'significance' level is too lenient for many situations in medicine.

A concentration ceiling for oxygen treatment   The single hospital experiment concerning oxygen treatment, that I cited earlier (p 122), provides an instructive lesson of the need to weigh consequences even when a relatively conservative risk level for Type I error is chosen. At the completion of that trial it was observed that the rate of irreversible RLF was reduced from 22 per cent under 'high' oxygen treatment to zero among infants assigned to 'low' oxygen management. The difference in outcomes was declared 'significant at about the 2 per cent level' and it was concluded that RLF-blindness could be *entirely* eliminated by a regimen of strict regulation of oxygen treatment.

The investigators advised that supplemental oxygen should be given only when there were unequivocal signs of need and that a gas concentration of 40 per cent (the ceiling used in the 'low' oxygen group) should not be exceeded. The 'under 40 per cent' advice was widely publicized, and there was general acceptance of the view that eye damage would not occur if the concentration of oxygen in incubators was carefully monitored and kept below the 'danger' level. This erroneous notion persisted for years despite a growing number of observations that RLF-blindness was not eradicated by these stringent restrictions of oxygen concentration and that early mortality was increased.

It is unlikely that a larger trial would have changed the verdict that 'low' oxygen reduces the risk of blindness (differences as large as the one observed would be expected to occur by chance only once in 50 trials involving about 40 babies in each group). However, the limits of what we may safely infer from zero occurrence of RLF in a sample of 40 infants might have been appreciated if the report had included the statement 'We are 95 per cent confident that the true risk of blindness after 'low' oxygen treatment lies between zero and 9 per cent.'

Estimates of this kind are called 'confidence intervals'; they indicate the range from the smallest to the largest effect of a treatment (or difference between treatments) with which the trial results are consistent. A 95 per cent confidence interval, for example, is the 2 standard deviation range surrounding the observed value; it expresses our conviction that the interval covers the (unknown) true value in 95 per cent of all possible samples (p 32). The additional information supplements the results of 'significance' testing and should be provided in complete reporting of trial results.

Trial size and claims of 'significance'

A report by Peto and co-workers noted that the size of a trial should be considered in assessing claims of 'statistical significance.' It was observed that for every trial that compares two treatments for cancer that are substantially different in effectiveness, there are probably five to ten 'negative' trials in progress (the compared therapies are essentially equal).

Numbers of trials that will be 'statistically significant'

Planned trial size	Expected outcomes. Proportions of 'events' in two treatments	No. of trials[a]	Decision[b]	
			'Non-significant'	'Significant'
About 250 'events' (enrollment of some hundreds of patients)	50% v. 50% (no real difference)	100	95 (right)	At least 5[c] (misleading)
	50% v. 33% (treatments really differ)	20	1 (misleading)	19[d] (right)
About 25 'events' (enrollment of some dozens of patients)	50% v. 50% (no real difference)	1000	950 (right)	At least 50[c] (misleading)
	50% v. 33% (treatments really differ)	200	150 (misleading)	50[d] (right)

[a] Numbers of such trials in progress throughout the world postulated by Peto's group.
[b] Given the postulated numbers, approximately how many will be declared 'nonsignificant', and how many 'significant' at $P \leq 0.05$?
[c] Even the most rigorously designed, executed and analyzed studies have a 1-in-20 chance of a false positive result with α set at $P \leq 0.05$. The less rigorous the study, the greater the chance of a false positive; in practice 10 per cent or more of all studies yield such false positives (at $P \leq 0.05$).
[d] A reduction from 50 per cent to 33 per cent mortality has a very good chance of being detected (19 out of 20) in a trial in which hundreds are randomized and about 250 of them die, but the chances are only 1 out of 4 that a difference of this size will be recognized in a small trial in which dozens are randomized and about 25 succumb.
(Taken from Peto and co-workers)

Given this situation, a few reasonable numbers were postulated and three conclusions were suggested from the projections. First, a large proportion of reports of 'statistically significant' treatment differences in small trials are misleading: differences of the size predicted do not exist. Second, if a small trial compares a new treatment that is so effective that it prevents one third of the deaths that occur under a control regimen, the study will probably fail to reach 'statistical significance'. Finally, a serious bias arises because most of the interesting therapeutic questions are being studied simultaneously by many investigators. Any trials, large or small, in which patients given the new therapy fare significantly better will be published and publicized. The studies that find no difference will rarely receive wide attention, especially if the numbers of enrolled patients are small.

The inevitable bias, the report concluded, can be circumvented to some extent by restricting attention to medical trials so large that they would be published whether or not an important outcome difference was observed.

Publication decisions

... There's this desert prison, see, with an old prisoner, resigned to his life, and a young one just arrived. The young one talks constantly of escape, and, after a few months, he makes a break. He's gone a week, and then he's brought back by the guards. He's half dead, crazy with hunger and thirst. He describes how awful it was to the old prisoner. The endless stretches of sand, no oasis, no signs of life anywhere. The old prisoner listens for a while, then says, 'Yep. I know. I tried to escape myself, twenty years ago.' The young prisoner says, 'You did? Why didn't you tell me, all these months I was planning my escape? Why didn't you let me know it was impossible?' And the old prisoner shrugs, and says, 'So who publishes negative results?'

Jeffrey Hudson

Publishing only 'significant' results

Theodore D. Sterling of the University of Cincinnati examined some of the issues concerning the publication of experimental results. He reviewed research reports in psychology research journals and found that of 294 articles using statistical tests, only 8 did not attain the 5 per cent 'significance' level. This evidence suggested that a fixed level of 'significance' was adopted as a criterion for submitting or accepting reports for publication. The practice, he noted, leads to unanticipated consequences.

When research that yields 'non significant' results is not published, the study may be repeated many times by investigators who are unaware of the previous efforts. Eventually, by chance, a 'statistically significant' result occurs—a Type I error—and this replication is published. Readers approach each report in a prestigious journal with the expectation that the results are 'statistically significant', but they should consider the possibility that a selection may have taken place. Among a set of similar experiments, the one that yielded large differences by chance had an artifically enhanced opportunity to come to their attention in print. Before readers can make an intelligent decision about what is published, they must have some information concerning the distribution of outcomes of similar experiments or at least some assurance that a similar test has never been performed. Since the needed information is unobtainable, the subscribers are in a quandary.

One thing is clear, Sterling observed: the risk of Type I error stated by the author should not be accepted at its face value. Since the general reluctance to publish negative results is easily confirmed by reading current medical articles, the cautionary advice is quite relevant.

'Significant' results in sub-classes

I have emphasized that in a focused trial the class of patients and an end point to be considered are clearly specified in advance; the quality of evidence is strengthened by limiting the problems associated with multiplicity.

The relationship between strength of evidence and multiplicity is described by Tukey in terms of the simple arithmetic of asking multiple ques-

Multiplicity of classes of patients and the probability of a 'significant' outcome

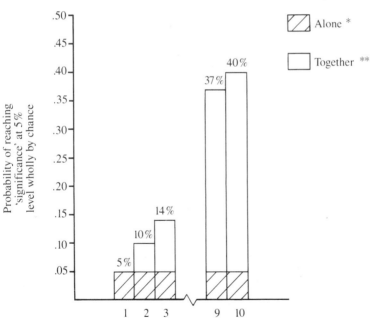

*For each class considered alone the probability of finding a 'significant' result is 100 per cent minus 95 per cent = 5 per cent

**For two classes the probability of finding at least one of the two results 'significant' is 100 per cent minus (95 per cent)$^2 \simeq 10$ per cent ... for ten classes the probability of finding at least one out of the 10 results 'significant' is 100 per cent minus (95 per cent)$^{10} \simeq 40$ per cent. (Based on compilation by Tukey)

tions and concentrating on the most favorable answers. In a hypothetical inquiry concerning the effect of a treatment that is perfectly neutral (totally without effect on any patient), as the classes of patients examined is increased, the likelihood of finding a 'significant' result in at least one of the subgroups purely by chance rises sharply. Thus, the evidence that for one class of patient, a broad inquiry has reached some specified level of 'statistical significance,' is much less powerful than the finding that pre-study specification of one class has reached exactly the same level of 'significance'.

Obviously, it is right for a physician to *want* to know about the behavior to be expected from a therapy when applied to his particular patient. But, Tukey points out, he cannot *expect* this. The national RLF study clearly indicated that such expectations are unrealistic. The limits of the generalizations that could be drawn from this time-consuming effort were quite narrow: RLF outcome was examined in 75 subclasses of patients, but questions concerning these 'passive' associations could only be resolved by further testing.

CONCEPTS OF STATISTICAL PROOF

'Significance' level as direct probability

A restriction in the concept of statistical proof can be seen by examining a distinction between finding an effect when we are given the causes and finding a cause when we are given effects. Statistician Richard B. Darlington of Cornell University points out that in the first situation we can make a prediction by calculating what is called 'direct' probability; for example, in coin tossing we compute the chances of 'heads' knowing the circumstances under which they are to occur. The second situation is an inverted one often found in medical experiments. We observe the event and ask, What is the probability that results from its occurrence in favor of any set of circumstances under which the same might have happened? The rules for calculating the latter so-called 'inverse' probability cannot be formulated without more information about the distribution of *causes*.

For instance, at the beginning of the national RLF trial, it was postulated (as in classical hypothesis testing) that oxygen curtailment would *not* reduce the risk of RLF by a specified amount. And it was necessary to *assume* that this hypothesis was true in order to calculate the probability of occurrence of the disorder in a group of babies treated in the new way. The no-important-reduction postulate was rejected because the observed reduction in the occurrence of blindness satisfied a pre-set 'significance' level (that is, *if* the hypothesis was, in fact, true, a reduction in RLF rate from 23 per cent to 7 per cent would be expected in only one of more than 100 trials of similar size). The reverse operation—calculating the probability that the no-important-reduction hypothesis was true on the basis of the actual occurrence of RLF under curtailed oxygen—could not be justified.

These convoluted sentences make the subtle but important distinction between forward and backward inference. A 'significance level' is a kind of direct probability: the probability of observing a certain type of event *if* the null hypothesis is true. Inverse probability concerns the probability that the null hypothesis is true if an event is observed. Darlington reminds us that in a purely scientific inquiry, we would really like to know the inverse probability, but we must normally be satisfied with knowing only the direct probability. To calculate the former, we must have some estimate of the probability of the hypothesis *before* knowing the data; this is called prior probability of the hypothesis. It is used in Bayesian analysis, a statistical approach based on a theorem proposed by Reverend Thomas Bayes, an eighteenth-century minister.

The Reverend Thomas Bayes' approach to inferences concerning hypotheses

('Subjective' or 'personal' probability)

What can be inferred about the probability of concurrence of a theorized cause and an outcome of interest from observations of associations between the two? For example, based on the observations in Melbourne hospitals reported in 1951 (p 19) concerning the co-incidence of 'free use of oxygen' and RLF, what is the probability of finding this association in *future* observations?

Oxygen Use	RLF Present	Absent	Total
Free use	a	b	$a+b$
	23	100	123
Conservative use	c	d	$c+d$
	4	54	58
Total	$a+c$	$b+d$	$a+b+c+d$
	27	154	191

(1) The relative frequency (or 'probability') of occurrence of the outcome of interest among those exposed to the theorized cause was

$$p = \frac{a}{a+b} = \frac{23}{123} = 0.19$$

This represents a 'conditional probability': the probability of RLF *on condition* of a history of 'free use of oxygen'. (Similarly, the probability of RLF on condition of a history of 'conservative use of oxygen' was $4 \div 58 = 0.07$)

(2) The relative frequency (or 'probability') of the theorized cause among those with the outcome of interest was

$$p = \frac{a}{a+c} = \frac{23}{27} = 0.85$$

The probability of a history of 'free use of oxygen' *on condition* that RLF is present.

Reverend Bayes proposed a theorem as a basis for inductive inference that has led to an approach often termed 'Bayesian statistics'. In the application of this method, Mainland explained, we seek to arrive at the conditional probability stated in (2) from the probabilities (relative frequencies) alone. For example,

(3) As noted in (1), the probability of RLF on condition of a history of 'free use of oxygen' was 0.19

(4) But those exposed to the 'free use of oxygen' constituted a given proportion of the total

$$p = \frac{a+b}{a+b+c+d} = \frac{123}{191} = 0.64$$

(5) Therefore, those with a history of 'free use of oxygen' who had RLF constituted
$$(3) \times (4) = 0.19 \times 0.64 = 0.12 \text{ of the total}$$

(6) All of the infants with RLF constituted

$$\frac{a+c}{a+b+c+d} = \frac{27}{191} = 0.14 \text{ of the total}$$

(7) As noted in (5), 0.12 of the total were exposed-affected, thus,

$$p = \frac{(5)}{(6)} = \frac{0.12}{0.14} = 0.85$$

The probability of finding a history of 'free use of oxygen' on the condition that RLF is present—the value obtained in (2).

(8) Bayes' Theorem takes this form to estimate the probability of concurrence of a theorized cause and an outcome of interest from observations of the two,

$$p = \frac{(1) \times (4)}{(6)} = \frac{0.19 \times 0.64}{0.14} = 0.85$$

On the assumption, belief, and hope that the observations on which these calculations are based represent a fair sample of 'all' infants at risk.

The 'free use of oxygen' is the hypothesis and RLF is a piece of data determined by observation. Note that the probability of 'free use of oxygen' was used in (4) as a relative frequency. It is what we would declare about an infant whom we knew to have a history of either 'free use of oxygen' or 'conservative use', if we knew the relative frequencies of these two histories, but *before* we knew about the presence or absence of RLF. It is therefore called a 'prior' or 'initial' probability in the classical approach. In Bayesian statistics, this is termed the 'prior probability of the hypothesis'—and in this sense it is a 'personal' probability, a statement of betting odds. (In fact, Bayes suggested that probability judgments based on mere hunches should be combined with probabilities based on relative frequencies.) Moreover, the conditional probabilities in (1), (6), and (8) are also considered 'personal' probabilities, in the sense that the frequencies and proportions favorable to total possibilities help form orderly and consistent opinions, rather than just any opinion. Statistical inference is modification of these opinions in the light of evidence, and Bayes' Theorem specifies how much modification should be made.
(Based on Mainland's exposition)

'Significance' as change in belief

The results of a trial with pragmatic emphasis also have some explanatory implications and our interest often extends beyond the purposes to which the results will be put. How can we describe the non-utilitarian aspect of conclusions drawn from a 'significance' level in some unambiguous way? Darlington suggests that the clearest interpretation is not as a *state* of belief but as a *change* in belief in a hypothesis. Words that imply this change are 'strengthen' or 'weaken'.

A result 'significant' at the 5 per cent level might be said to 'strengthen the alternative hypothesis' or to 'weaken the null hypothesis', depending on the interpreter's previous views. However, if an observer has no opinion before seeing the result, the outcome will produce a large change of personal view. In these circumstances, a term implying a state rather than a change of belief may be appropriate: 'the result confirms the experimental hypothesis at the 5 per cent level of significance' (and the antonym here is 'disconfirm').

'Not proven' verdict

The words used to describe 'non-significance' also need to be chosen carefully to avoid misunderstanding. R.W. Smithells of the University of Leeds has noted that English law insists that a prisoner is innocent until proven guilty. But the declaration at the end of a negative trial is less likely to mislead, he advised, when the rule of Scottish law is followed: a verdict of 'not proven' is permitted.

The latter terminology reminds us that failure to *demonstrate* differences does not prove that they are in fact negligible (p 119).

Practical interpretation

At the end of a pragmatic trial we envisage some practical action that will be taken when a verdict statement is made. Even when we decide that there is no important difference between compared treatments, practical considerations may lead to a decision in favor of the innovation. Such action is not determined solely on the basis of 'significance level' since we prefer treatments that are readily accepted by patients, easy to administer, and inexpensive. The move, then, from decisions made about the results of a clinical trial to individual value judgments made at the bedside needs to be examined if we are to understand the process by which a medical innovation is translated into something of social value.

In the next chapter, I propose to discuss how individuals (the physician and the patient) and communities faced with a problem of choice under uncertainty may go about deciding on a course of action that is consistent with individual basic judgements and preference.

I fear that I have spent so much time in this chapter on the 'ifs', 'ands', 'buts', and 'howevers' when making statistical inferences that I may have given a mistaken impression that an approach based on the science of chance is a very weak one. (Harry Truman once confessed that he was looking for a one-armed economist to provide him with a solution for the country's economic woes. All of his advisors hedged their remarks by saying, 'On the one hand ..., but on the other hand ...') But (if I can be permitted one last adversative conjunction) there is little need to sing the praises of the goddess of fortune. She is generous in her rewards to those who stick with the odds. It is possible to 'break the bank at Monte Carlo' by betting against the house and dismissing the laws of probability with a snap of the fingers, but don't bet your life on it.

> For we know in part, and we prophecy in part ...
> For now we see through a glass darkly; ...
> I *Corinthians* 9 and 12

11 Extrapolation of trial results

As the Renaissance in Europe was drawing to a close, some gamblers were caught up in the new spirit of inquiry. They became curious about the pattern of numbers that kept turning up in the fall of dice. Unable to answer their own questions about these seemingly fateful happenings, they approached some of the leading scientists of the day for help. A group of Italian gamblers met with an interested reception when they consulted Galileo. The busy astronomer-physicist found the gaming problems worthy of study, and he went on to write a treatise on die-throwing sometime between 1613 and 1623.

A short time later (ca 1654), history repeated itself in France. A famous gambler, the Chevalier de Méré, was perplexed about 'the problem of points in the die game'. He brought the questions to his friend, Blaise Pascal, the mathematical genius. Subsequently, Pascal and his correspondent, Pierre de Fermat, in a famous exchange of letters, developed a solution to the problem and they generalized the result in the form of tables that indicated how stakes should be divided in games between two players if they decide to quit at a moment when neither has definitely won. These 'beautiful ideas about games of chance' were admired by other mathematicians and led directly to the development of the theory of probability.

PRACTICAL ACTION IN THE FACE OF UNCERTAINTY

I find it interesting that the new theory arose in response to the needs of those who risked their fortunes daily on actions taken in the face of uncertainty. And considering the number of parallels between gambling and medicine that I have drawn on, I am not surprised that the regular workings of the laws of chance had been anticipated in the mid 1500s by a physician, Giralomo Cardano.

State of nature

The theory of probability may be defined as the logic of degrees of belief concerning the occurrence of uncertain events. But what do we mean by

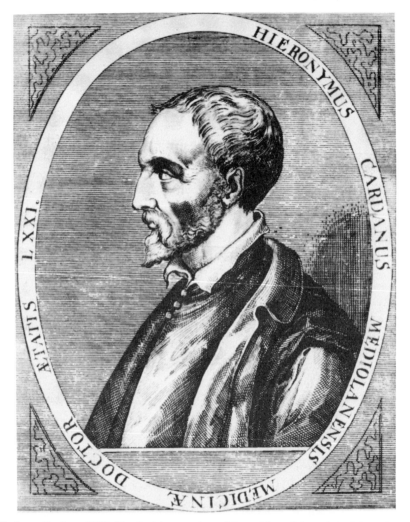

Giralomo Cardano (1501–76: physician, mathematician, philosopher, and gambler) was the first to calculate a probability correctly (*ca* 1563 or 1564). In an obscure text on games of chance (*Liber de Ludo Aleae*, The Book on Games of Chance, that appeared after his death), he discussed equiprobability, mathematical expectation, reasoning concerning the mean, frequency tables for dice probabilities, additive properties of probabilities, and the question of how many trials are required to give a player an even chance of winning: for example, to throw a given point total in a game of dice.

uncertainty? Recall that there are two kinds of uncertain events. One is due to the kind of randomness exemplified by the fall of honest dice considered by Pascal and Fermat. The other kind of uncertainty arises when the abstract calculation of odds concerning *equi*probable events does not work. The latter are the situations in which we do not know which laws of randomness apply. In statistical terminology the 'state of nature' is unknown. How do we develop a betting strategy for a game involving 'loaded' dice in which one result is favored? As already noted, here we are obliged to undertake a series of observations to estimate the state of nature, but we are immediately confronted by the issue of deciding when we have made 'enough' observations. The judgment depends on the cost of each throw of the dice and the cost of making a wrong decision.

Obviously, we can never be certain about the state of nature no matter how many observations we record concerning the behavior of the dice. For example, it is possible, although highly unlikely, that honest dice will turn up 'seven' in a very high proportion of a hundred consecutive throws. It is also possible, and improbable, that dice weighted to favor 'seven' will turn up 'three' in the majority of one hundred plays.

To evaluate the chances of being led astray by rare results, we turn to the theory of probability. But action-oriented decisions (such as 'our estimate of the state of nature is good enough to place a bet', 'the odds offered are satisfactory', and '$100 is a reasonable wager') cannot be undertaken rationally until we have considered some additional 'facts of life' having to do with values. It is just this kind of situation that faces the physician who must decide on a practical course of action in the best interest of his individual patient.

Disciplined approach to action-oriented decisions

The decision problem under uncertainty is not unique in gambling and in medicine. Recent years have seen the development of practical strategies for balancing risks and benefits when making decisions in states of doubt. These have evolved into the discipline of decision analysis, that has found wide application in fields ranging from military strategy to public health.

On being right or wrong   Before discussing the analytic approach to decision making, I should mention that we tend to have unrealistic expectations about the predictions used to make decisions, particularly when the resultant actions produce irreversible effects on our everyday lives. From our perspective as patients, the overriding concern is the correctness of decisions. Alan R. Shapiro of Stanford University, however, points out that we need to distinguish a decision from the evidence on which that decision is based.

In evaluating predictive ability, we must recognize that a final decision is the result of a number of considerations, such as various value assessments and outcomes whose meaning is unique to a particular patient. What is needed in judging predictions, Shapiro notes, is a method for assessing the accuracy of the probabilities asserted, not an all-or-none scoring of decisions as right or wrong.

Frustration and confusion about decisions based on before-the-event predictions come up frequently in clinical medicine. When a surgeon declares before an operation that the mortality risk of the procedure is only 1 per cent and the patient dies on the first postoperative day, the anger of the family and friends is understandable. But it cannot be concluded that the pre-event probability was wrong; without more evidence, we can only say that an improbable event occurred.

Formulation of a decision problem when faced with conditions of uncertainty

1 Specify the viable options available for gathering information, for experimentation, and for action.

2 Specify the events that may possibly occur.

3 Arrange the information that may be acquired in chronologic order, and the choices that may be made with the passage of time.

4 Decide on preferences about the consequences resulting from various courses of action that can be taken (preferences for consequences numerically scaled in terms of utility values).

5 Make a judgment concerning the chances that any particular uncertain event will occur (judgment about uncertainty numerically scaled in terms of probability).

(From Howard Raiffa of Harvard University)

DECISION ANALYSIS

The development of decision theory has provided an analytic guide to the way in which we go about making value decisions in everyday life. The approach lends itself to a logical analysis of decisions in medicine.

First, we need to quantify information and preferences and then proceed in an orderly sequence. Decision analysts advise that a rational choice of treatment requires that we define outcomes and the probabilities of outcomes and that we make some estimate of the values or utilities of the state of health that constitute the outcomes (utility is a numerical measure of worth). Moreover, judgment should be based on the state of each patient as an individual rather than on the disease label.

Decision theory in medicine

Definitions of some terms

Decision theory: a theory of decision functions which assumes that it is possible to attach a measure of worth or value to any state of health.

Decision function: action (decided in advance) that will be undertaken as a function of possible outcomes. Ideally, we should like to be able to express possible medical treatments as a decision function whose independent variables are the possible sets of indicants that might occur on any one occasion.

Indicant: any piece of evidence relevant to the probability that a disease is present.

Event: a feature of the state of the patient referring to his state of health.

Event space: the state of a patient is conceived as specifiable, in principle, by a sequence of measurements some of which might be impracticable by existing methods. Each measurement is regarded as a coordinate and the sequence of measurements thus corresponds to a point in multidimensional space called 'event space'.

Utility: the concept of utility (in a sense borrowed from economics where the worth of outcomes is measured numerically; each outcome is given a single number called its utility) is useful in defining objectives in medicine. A doctor attempts to increase each patient's utility, but has no certainty, only a probability of achieving this. Thus it is more accurate to speak of expected utility. The expected utility is the sum of the probabilities of the utilities of all mutually exclusive outcomes. The calculation requires the estimation of the utilities of the states of health of the patient, and the combination of these with the costs of the course of action. Utility is expressed as a mathematical variable or function corresponding to the state of the world for a person. It is assumed that if a person's behaviors and choices satisfy certain compelling postulates the individual will behave as if he/she

–has subjective probability estimates about the state of the world

–has associated a real function with possible states of the world

–wishes to maximize the expected value of the function.

Quasi-utility: when some relevant utilities are too difficult to estimate, it is of value to define some function of probabilities of the more readily estimated utilities whose expectation is estimated instead. Such a function is called a 'quasi-utility'.

Utile: any unit in terms of which utilities could be measured.

Cost: negative contribution to utility; expressed in financial terms or in terms of danger, anxiety or pain to the patient.

Principle of rationality: the maximization of the mathematical expectation of utility, by choice of actions.

Rationality: consistency of choice, and adherence to the principle of rationality.

(Taken from Card and Good)

Diagnostic process

Medical activity, from first examination to active treatment, has been envisioned by W.I. Card and I.J. Good of the University of Glasgow as a sequence of decisions under the general heading of diagnosis. The indicators of disease (called 'indicants') are obtained by questions, laboratory tests, and other procedures at each stage in the overall diagnostic process. A collection of indicants is chosen by the doctor and this selection (among a number of possible sets) decides the next move in the methodic approach.

A medical decision model

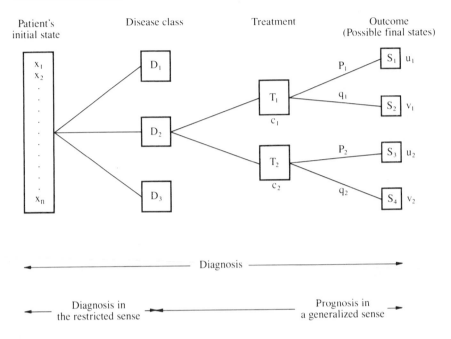

The diagnostic process, Card and Good explain, consists of eliciting a set of indicants from a patient and, on the basis of these, allocating the sufferer to a disease class. Choice of treatment T_1 costs c_1 and with probabilities p_1 and q_1, respectively, produces gains in health utility u_1 and v_1. Similarly, treatment T_2 costs c_2 and with probabilities p_2 and q_2, respectively, produces gains in health utility of u_2 and v_2.

Diagnosis may be regarded as following the branches along a decision tree. The course may be compared to the diagram of a game in which the doctor chooses a move at each stage of the match, and an opponent (the goddess of fortune) chooses a play. The physician's overall search strategy is formed by decisions based on current knowledge, not the whole tree which represents all possible games that could be played.

Gain in utility   The rules for the choice of indicants will depend on the initial probabilities of various possible diseases, the expected utilities of their treatments, and on the costs or negative utilities of tests and treatments. A doctor attempts to increase each patient's utility, and the objective is achieved by the choices that are under his control.

In the early stages the gain in utility is indirect: a gain in certainty which, it is hoped, will lead to the best treatment. The estimate of the probability that a specific disease is present may be calculated by Bayes' Theorem

Benefits and costs of treatment choices

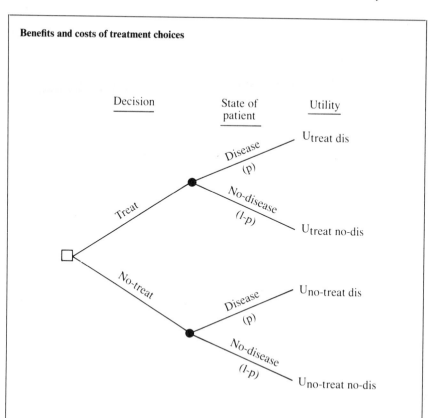

In this hypothetical example, the choice to be made by the physician ($\square$) is whether or not to administer positive pressure to a baby with hyaline membrane disease (treat or no-treat). With either choice, chance will 'decide' ($\bullet$) that the infant either has the disease (with probability p) or does not (probability $1 - p$).

Four possible outcomes are represented by the terminal branches of the tree, and each has a certain utility value (e.g. $U_{treat\ dis}$, the utility of administering positive-pressure treatment to patients with hyaline membrane disease). If the four utilities are measured in consistent units (e.g. duration of life*, parental value terms, societal value terms, dollars, ...), the values of the outcomes can be compared and ordered.

On the assumption that the benefit of positive pressure is restricted to patients with hyaline membrane disease, net benefit can be expressed as the difference between the utility of administering treatment to affected babies and the utility of withholding treatment in the same class of infants:

(1) Net benefit $= U_{treat\ dis} - U_{no\text{-}treat\ dis}$

The cost may be expressed as the difference between the utility of avoiding treatment in unaffected babies and the utility of administering treatment in the unaffected class of infants:

(2) Net cost $= U_{\text{no-treat no-dis}} - U_{\text{treat no-dis}}$

The expected value (EV) of the two courses of action may be calculated as follows:

(3) $EV_{\text{treat}} = (p) U_{\text{treat dis}} + (1-p) U_{\text{treat no-dis}}$

(4) and $EV_{\text{no-treat}} = (p) U_{\text{no-treat dis}} + (1-p)U_{\text{no-treat no-dis}}$

A rational choice is the course of action with the higher expected value. When the expected values of the two courses of action are equal, it is rational to remain indifferent. From the above expressions, the probability value at the indifference point is derived as follows:

Equation (3) = Equation (4)

and solving for p (the probability at the indifference point),

$$p = \frac{U_{\text{no-treat no-dis}} - U_{\text{treat no-dis}}}{U_{\text{treat dis}} - U_{\text{no-treat dis}} + U_{\text{no-treat no-dis}} - U_{\text{treat no-dis}}}$$

If the probability of the disease in a given patient is greater than the probability at the indifference point, treatment is rational; if the probability of the disease is less than the 'indifferent' value, withholding treatment would seem to be rational.

(Adapted from the arguments of S.F. Pauker and J.P. Kassirer of Tufts University)

*The utilities of positive-pressure treatment and no treatment must take into account the probability of survival with complications (e.g. blindness, brain damage, ...) under these two courses of action.

(p 135) for conditional probability (using prior information about the frequency of diseases and the accumulation of indicants).

The cost-benefit trade-off of therapeutic decisions may also be calculated by assigning numerical values to probabilities and to utilities.

Function of randomized trials   When viewed from this structured perspective, the function of randomized clinical trials in medicine emerges in a clear light. The formal exercises provide the basis for predictions of the outcomes following specific treatments. The hard-to-obtain information is used by physicians in everyday management decisions for individual patients, but it should be understood that the translation of these medical judgments into practical actions requires that patients (or their surrogates) make value judgments.

Subjective judgments

The question of whether utilities should be regarded as belonging to the theory of probability may be argued at some length. Howard Raiffa of

> The player on the other side is hidden from us. We know that his play is always fair, just, and patient. But also we know, to our cost, that he never overlooks a mistake, or makes the smallest allowance for ignorance. To the man who plays well, the highest stakes are paid, with that sort of overflowing generosity with which the strong show delight in strength. And one who plays ill is checkmated—without haste, but without remorse.
>
> T.H. Huxley

Harvard University has pointed out that the subjectivists (those who hold with Reverend Bayes) wish to introduce intuitive judgments and feelings directly into the formal analysis of a decision problem. The objectivists argue that these subjective aspects are best left out of the formal analysis and should be used only to bridge the gap between the real world and the objective results obtained in the use of a formal model.

Despite the philosophical debates, there can be little doubt that a patient's subjective impressions of the state of the world cannot be ignored. And the analytic approach of decision theory forces us to make a distinction between the roles of the two participants in medical decisions: the doctor and the patient (or a surrogate).

We assume from observing ordinary human behavior in a world full of risks that rational persons act as if they had sets of probabilities and utilities that determine their choices of action at every turn in their lives. The principle of rationality is followed when there is a consistency of choices that increase the expectation of gain in utility. In a medical setting, it is reasonable to expect that when doctors provide patients with estimates of the probable outcomes of interventions, the sufferers will make rational decisions about the options that are available to them.

The seeds of misunderstanding lie buried in the phrase 'gain in utility'. Clearly, this function can only be defined and weighted in meaningful terms by patients and their families. Not surprisingly, private and public values are not always identical, and the value scales of the medical profession may be quite different from those of both patients and communities. The inevitable conflicts lead to some of the ethical problems that I will discuss in the next chapter.

Halting acceptance of formal methods

It would be misleading to leave the impression that physicians have adopted the reasoning of decision theorists to guide decision making at the bedside. The development of formal methods for the quantification of judgment to replace traditional intuitive approaches in medicine has been halting. The principal difficulty is that of making numerical estimates of the utilities of possible outcomes of medical interventions. I believe the resistance stems from our reluctance to make what seems to be cold and scheming statements about the *prospect* of negative utilities associated with horrendous possibilities like blindness, brain damage, and death. On the other hand, the emotional blocks are surmounted when we are asked to make the same cost estimates after the fact: the numbers are supplied for tort claims and insurance awards.

Additionally, the sensitive question concerning the extent to which medical practice should be based on economic principles is not easily discussed. I believe, however, that we cannot ignore the experience in other fields concerned with our lives and well-being; there has been a fairly general shift from haphazard methods to disciplined systems for decision making. Moreover, the benefits of systematic approaches in medicine are testable. Improvement may be measured in formal comparisons by the gain in utility of the state of health of patients and by the cost of achieving a change.

WIDESPREAD MEDICAL ACTION

I have said that we may look to the results of randomized trials for guidance concerning probable outcomes of treatment in a specific patient and that we may estimate the cost of our errors in relying on this information. The potential cost mounts with the treatment of large numbers of additional patients; the price of wide extrapolation of a misleading result may turn out to be quite high (as we saw in the example of the national RLF trial). Thus, if the results of a bedside trial seem to be important, independent confirmatory trials are highly desirable.

Recommendations for repeated demonstrations

R.A. Fisher commented, 'In order to assert that a natural phenomenon is experimentally demonstrated we need, not an isolated record, but a reliable method of procedure ... we may say that a phenomenon is experimentally demonstrable when we know how to conduct an experiment which will rarely fail to give us a statistically significant result [i.e. a result in the same direction and of similar magnitude].' This caution was expressed many years ago in reference to agricultural studies in which the experimenter was able to exert much more control over extraneous influences than in the highly unstable conditions found in medical settings.

The need for replications of clinical trials was underscored by Mainland early in the history of the use of these formats: the only way to learn something about the safety of our numerical findings, he noted, is by more extensive exploration under other conditions, in other places, and at other times.

Evaluation of social effectiveness

An additional argument can be made for cautious, progressively staged extrapolation of the results of treatment trials rather than single-step widespread applications. The reasoning was advanced by Halfdan Mahler, the Director-General of the World Health Organization. He pointed out that health development is essentially a political and social process that should start off with the acceptance of the social function of health. Technical developments need to be applied in harmony with this social function.

In many communities the value of expensive treatments can be seriously questioned if measured in terms of their impact on improving the health status of the populations. Governments and people have a right to an objective assessment of medical innovations. This implies that critical evaluation of an intervention entails not only tests of effectiveness in modifying the course of disease but also controlled community trials to determine acceptance and to explore methods of implementing the new approach. The last step is one of evaluating social effectiveness.

Activism versus the slow pace

I have now proposed many roadblocks to the speedy and widespread use of the potential cures developed by modern biomedical research. But it must be obvious that these overly cautious views are not shared by all who are engaged in the search for ways and means to reduce human suffering. In fact, there is a fairly sharp division between two ideologies. Sackett has dubbed the adversaries as the 'evangelists' and the 'snails'.

Evangelists In the presence of an on-going toll of disability and untimely death, the evangelists conclude that pre-existing evidence plus common sense demand intervention *now* even in the absence of experiments to test whether extrapolations from optimistic pre-clinical studies will, in fact, alter risk.

This attitude is bolstered by public clamor for rapid dissemination of new biomedical knowledge, and for conversion of this information into forms directly useful in the control of major diseases. Legislators demand a visible payoff on the investment of public funds in medical research. The activist viewpoint has been called the 'Lyndon Johnson doctrine', after a speech in which he chided the American research community for its alleged failure to translate the findings of laboratory investigation speedily into practice.

Additionally, the evangelistic view tends to see rational decisions as 'terminal': a particular hypothesis is to be acted upon without further experiments.

Snails The methodologists are the snails. They are wed to a series of criteria and strategies that, if rigorously applied, will increase the likelihood that the ultimate action is 'correct'. They insist that interventions must meet scientific and political criteria before they are widely implemented. And this school of thought is inclined to see rational decisions as 'sequential': a sequential decision is a judgment to perform further particular experiments.

Modern dangers   Paradoxically, one can make a stronger argument for the snail's pace in the present era of rapid increase in the volume of biomedical information than in the leisurely past. This incongruity arises from the fact that the magnitude of the consequences of error has escalated so sharply in recent years. The harmless nostrums of the past have been replaced by exceedingly powerful agents, and the means for broadcasting information about treatments have become very efficient.

The image of the physician as a romantic warrior armed with a sword to conquer disease is outdated. The modern doctor may be likened to a weapons specialist manning the push-button console of a missile launcher. Modern conditions call for cautious tactics: limited forays and carefully planned battles against ignorance concerning medical matters.

Simple concern for the public interest dictates that we cannot ignore Claude Bernard's maxim: science teaches us to doubt and, in ignorance, to refrain.

Abatement of loss

The wary approach to choice under conditions of uncertainty is based on a consideration of the worst that can happen. One principle that has been suggested is called the 'minimax average loss rule': pick that strategy for which the largest average loss is as small as possible.

Patients must consider not only how often they may 'lose', but the magnitude of the loss. In gambling terms they must weigh the size of the risk against the size of their 'bankroll'.

The thalidomide disaster   The issues were highlighted by the thalidomide tragedy that began when this drug was introduced in West Germany in 1957. It was regarded as a safe and useful medication, especially in the treatment of nausea during pregnancy. In late 1961, the West German Minister of Health issued a statement warning pregnant women not to take the drug; it was found to be associated with malformations (seal-like deformities of the limbs) that occurred in thousands of babies born to treated women throughout the world. Although the agent was not released for general use in the United States, $2\frac{1}{2}$ million tablets were made available to 1267 American physicians for informal clinical 'investigation'.

Legal brake on drug certification   As a direct result of the thalidomide experience, the Kefauver-Harris Amendment to the US Pure Food and

---

Phases of drug evaluation in the United States

Food and Drug Administration Guidelines

Phase I   *Initial administration of a drug to human subjects.*
Following the satisfactory completion of studies in animal models, a new drug is administered to a few volunteers (usually healthy persons) in order to determine the metabolic transformation and excretion of the compound, and to estimate levels of tolerance. This step is followed by dose-ranging studies for safety and, in some cases, pilot trials of efficacy are carried out in selected patients.

Phase II   *Early controlled clinical trials designed to evaluate efficacy and relative safety.*
Relatively small numbers of patients are enrolled in closely monitored studies (the numbers seldom involve more than 100–200 individuals who receive the new agent). Drugs considered to be effective and safe then enter Phase III.

Phase III   *Expanded controlled and uncontrolled trials.*
These studies are performed after efficacy has been tentatively established. The stage is focused on gathering additional evidence of efficacy, safety, and tolerance; and on the definition of adverse effects. Hundreds, sometimes thousands, of patients are enrolled in Phase III studies conducted in outpatient clinics and hospital wards (an effort is made to approximate the environments in which the new agent will be used). Drugs which complete Phase III studies satisfactorily are released for use by practising physicians.

Phase IV   *Post-marketing clinical trials.*
Additional studies to investigate the frequency rates of adverse reactions and specific pharmacologic effects are conducted in the field. Large-scale, long-term surveillance to determine the effect of a drug on morbidity and mortality is carried out in some instances to supplement and confirm pre-release data.

Drug Laws was passed in 1962. For the first time legal regulations set out the formal steps to be taken in testing the safety and efficacy of a new drug for human use.

This law played an important role in damping the exuberance that characterized the proliferation of new drugs in the years following the spectacular successes of penicillin and polio vaccine. The rate at which new drugs were released for general use slowed abruptly, and there has been much debate about these developments. Many have concluded (especially as the memory of the thalidomide tragedy fades) that the restrictive regulations must be relaxed because they hamper the development of 'effective' drugs and slow medical progress. An advisory committee examined the charges against strict regulations in the United States and found that there had been a worldwide slowing of new drug development. The advisors concluded, however, that deceleration was 'mainly the result of limitations of scientific understanding of biological actions in disease processes'.

Coordinated advance in medicine

From the arguments that I have made in this book it should be clear that I cast my lot with the snails. If more attention is paid to the clarification of goals than to the perfection of means, the rate of innovative change in medicine will, indeed, be slower than it has been in the recent past. In the words of Lewis Mumford, 'A pace of change might [be] established in relation to human need. Instead of rapid advances, on the basis of uncoordinated knowledge in specialized areas, there [will be] the possibility of a slower, but better coordinated advance that [does] justice to the processes, functions, and purposes of life.'

12 The ethics of human experimentation

Since the time of Hippocrates, Western physicians have taken an oath in which they swear to protect their patients 'from whatever is deleterious and mischievous'. As it turned out in much of the past, common treatments were neither specifically nor intentionally injurious: most were harmless palliatives. Even when doctors used highly lethal agents like mercury and arsenic as supposed remedies, injury and death occurred on a relatively small scale if for no other reason than the fact that few could afford professional services. Nevertheless, the long list of truly assaultive therapies that were available and the persistence of barbarous practices like copious blood-letting are quite incredible.

REACTION TO EXUBERANT TREATMENT

In 1835, Pierre Charles Alexandre Louis, of Paris, used the numerical method to bolster his argument that exsanguinations were of little value in the treatment of pneumonia. Louis' influence led his American pupil, the elder Oliver Wendell Holmes, to declare, in 1860, that nearly all drugs then in use should be thrown '... into the sea where it would be better for mankind and all the worse for the fishes'. In the latter part of the nineteenth century there was a trend away from exuberant therapies. The movement was led by the new Viennese school of 'therapeutic nihilism'. A leading exponent said, 'While we can diagnose and describe disease, we dare not expect by any manner of means to cure it.'

A break with the past

The development of the germ theory of disease only one hundred years ago was responsible for a qualitative break with the past. There was now hope for specific treatments. The search began for what Paul Ehrlich—the founder of the Institute for Experimental Therapy in 1899 at Frankfurt, Germany—called 'magic bullets' to eradicate the agents of disease without injuring the host. For the first time, an observer commented, 'an average

Seventeenth century treatment

At eight o'clock on Monday morning of February 2, 1685, King Charles II of England was being shaved in his bedroom. With a sudden cry he fell backward and had a violent convulsion. He became unconscious, rallied once or twice, and, after a few days, died. Doctor Scarburgh, one of the twelve or fourteen physicians called to treat the stricken king, recorded the efforts made to cure the patient.

As the first step in treatment the king was bled to the extent of a pint from a vein in his right arm. Next his shoulder was cut into and the incised area was 'cupped' to suck out an additional eight ounces of blood. After this, the drugging began. An emetic and purgative were administered, and soon after a second purgative. This was followed by an enema containing antimony, sacred bitters, rock salt, mallow leaves, violets, beetroot, camomile flowers, fennel seed, linseed, cinnamon, cardamom seed, saphron, cochineal, and aloes. The enema was repeated in two hours and a purgative given. The king's head was shaved and a blister raised on his scalp. A sneezing powder of hellebore root was administered, and also a powder of cowslip flowers 'to strengthen his brain'.

The cathartics were repeated at frequent intervals and interspersed with a soothing drink composed of barley water, liquorice, and sweet almond. Likewise white wine, absinthe, and anise were given, as also were extracts of thistle leaves, mint, rue, and angelica. For external treatment a plaster of Burgundy pitch and pigeon dung was applied to the king's feet. The bleeding and purging continued, and to the medicaments were added melon seeds, manna, slippery elm, black cherry water, an extract of flowers of lime, lily of the valley, peony, lavender, and dissolved pearls. Later came gentian root, nutmeg, quinine, and cloves.

The king's condition did not improve, indeed it grew worse, and in the emergency forty drops of extract of human skull were administered to allay convulsions. A rallying dose of Raleigh's antidote was forced down the king's throat; this antidote contained an enormous number of herbs and animal extracts. Finally bezoar stone was given. 'Then,' said Scarburgh, 'Alas! after an ill-fated night his serene majesty's strength seemed exhausted to such a degree that the whole assembly of physicians lost all hope and became despondent: still so as not to appear to fail in doing their duty in any detail, they brought into play the most active cordial.' As a sort of grand summary to this pharmaceutical debauch, a mixture of Raleigh's antidote, pearl julep, and ammonia was forced down the throat of the dying king.

(Noted by H.W. Haggard)

patient treated by an average practitioner could expect a better than fifty-fifty chance of improvement'.

Deep-seated suspicion

The recently developed formal methods to evaluate specific interventions are intended, as I have discussed, to increase these odds. But deeply rooted fears of medicine's ancient excesses persist, and suspicions are rekindled by unfortunate incidents that are a reminder of the misguided past.

The phrase 'human experimentation' is beset with some dreadful connotations. The expression conjures up the image of demented doctors working in a chamber of horrors, and the destructive myth is exploited in lurid novels and in horror films.

FORMAL CODES OF MEDICAL ETHICS

A model for these frightening representations was provided by the all too real criminal behavior of physicians in the concentration camps of Nazi Germany during World War II who committed murders, tortures, and other atrocities in the name of medical science. Twenty doctors were tried for these crimes following the war. In the decision at the end of the trial, the panel of judges set out ten principles that must be observed in the conduct of human experimentation in order to satisfy moral, ethical, and legal concepts. These principles became known as the Nuremberg Code of 1947.

An international code

The Declaration of Helsinki, a formal code of ethics for the guidance of doctors in clinical research, was adopted by the World Medical Association in 1964, and the recommendations were extended in 1975. The revised code ('Helsinki II') took into account various considerations that arose in the intervening years. The Council for International Organizations of Medical Sciences and the World Health Organization, which played an active part in the preparation of the statement, indicated that the text would be subject to periodic review in the light of criticisms and comments. In September 1981 the Council endorsed a set of guidelines to suggest how the general principles of Helsinki II might be applied in the special circumstances of many technologically developing countries.

Proliferation of codes

It is notable that a number of codes and guidelines have been drafted, over the years following World War II, by such organizations as the American Medical Association, the American Psychological Association, the American Academy of Pediatrics, the British Medical Research Council, the British Paediatric Association, the National Institutes of Health, and the Association of American Medical Colleges (and the list is not complete). Jay Katz of Yale Law School has pointed out that the proliferation of such declarations testifies to the difficulty of developing a set of rules that do not have what may be called 'open texture'. By necessity, the canons have had to be succinctly worded, and their meaning has been subject to a variety of interpretations. Significant discrepancies between the codes also have helped to sow confusion.

Limited usefulness of general exhortation Katz opined that as long as these precepts remain unelaborated tablets of exhortation to promote ideal practices, they will, at best, have limited usefulness in guiding daily behavior of investigators.

The international code of ethics for biomedical research

Helsinki II

Basic principles in the Declaration of Helsinki, revised and extended by the Twenty-Ninth World Medical Assembly in Tokyo, 1975.

1   Biomedical research involving human subjects must conform to generally accepted scientific principles and should be based on adequately performed laboratory and animal experimentation and on a thorough knowledge of the scientific literature.

2   The design and performance of each experimental procedure involving human subjects should be clearly formulated in an experimental protocol which should be transmitted to a specially appointed independent committee for consideration, comment and guidance.

3   Biomedical research involving human subjects should be conducted only by scientifically qualified persons and under the supervision of a clinically competent medical person. The responsibility for the human subject must always rest with a medically qualified person and never rest on the subject of the research even though the subject has given his or her consent.

4   Biomedical research involving human subjects cannot legitimately be carried out unless the importance of the objective is in proportion to the inherent risk to the subject.

5   Every biomedical research project involving human subjects should be preceded by careful assessment of predictable risks in comparison with foreseeable benefits to the subject or to others. Concern for the interest of the subject must always prevail over the interests of science and society.

6   The right of the research subject to safeguard his or her integrity must always be respected. Every precaution should be taken to respect the privacy of the subject and to minimize the impact of the study on the subject's physical and mental integrity and on the personality of the subject.

7   Doctors should abstain from engaging in research projects involving human subjects unless they are satisfied that the hazards involved are believed to be predictable. Doctors should cease any investigation if the hazards are found to outweigh the potential benefits.

8   In the publication of the results of his or her research, the doctor is obliged to preserve the accuracy of the results. Reports on experimentation not in accordance with the principles laid down in this Declaration should not be accepted for publication.

9   In any research on human beings, each potential subject must be adequately informed of the aims, methods, anticipated benefits and potential hazards of the study and the discomfort it may entail. He or she should be informed that he or she is at liberty to abstain from participation in the study and that he or she is free to withdraw his or her consent to participation at any time. The doctor should then obtain the subject's freely-given informed consent, preferably in writing.

10   When obtaining informed consent for the research project the doctor should be particularly cautious if the subject is in a dependent relationship to him or her or may consent under duress. In that case the informed consent should be obtained by a doctor who is not engaged in the investigation and who is completely independent of this official relationship.

11   In the case of legal incompetence, informed consent should be obtained from the legal guardian in accordance with national legislation. Where physical or mental incapacity makes it impossible to obtain informed consent, or when the subject is a minor, permission from the responsible relative replaces that of the subject in accordance with national legislation.

12   The research protocol should always contain a statement of the ethical considerations involved and should indicate that the principles enunciated in the present Declaration are complied with.

Justice Holmes once warned, 'General propositions do not decide concrete cases. The decision will depend on a judgment or intuition more subtle than any articulated major premise.' Indeed, the attempts to develop statutes for regulating the activities of medical experimentalists have been unsatisfactory; the ethical declarations are not legal documents. A British bill dealing with some aspects of experimentation in children was described by one Queen's Counsel as demonstrating the 'clumsiness of the law as a means of fine control of human endeavor'.

Failure of self-regulation

The promulgation of various codes of ethics may be viewed as tacit recognition within the medical and behavioral science professions that self-regulation by investigators could not be relied on to control research practices. However, headline scandals played the major role in focusing public attention on the issues.

Scandals The most widely publicized incident occurred in 1963 when two respected scientists who were studying the immune response to cancer injected live malignant cells into a number of aged patients in a chronic disease hospital without first obtaining the patients' consent.

More recently, the press disclosed a study conducted by the Public Health Service (PHS) which had been underway since the 1930s. A group of black men with syphilis had been kept under observation to record the 'natural' course of the disease. During the early years of inaction the observational study—the longest of its kind in medical history—was rationalized by the investigators on grounds that the drugs then available were toxic and only marginally effective. Moreover, when the study was undertaken, the PHS officials were unable to obtain funds for the accepted treatment of the day in an impoverished rural county. Despite the fact that in 1945 penicillin became available as a safe, cheap, and dramatically effective cure for syphilis, the no-treatment observations continued. It has been presumed, with good reason, that some men died of the disease who could have been cured.

Prior review

Such disgraceful episodes and other less widely publicized examples of unrestrained investigative activities led to the development of procedures to implement the general principles stated in the codes of ethics. The move began in the United States with a memorandum from Surgeon-General William H. Steward, dated February 1966, that was sent to the heads of institutions conducting research with Public Health Service grants. The requirement of prior review had been in effect since 1953 for clinical research conducted within the Clinical Center in Bethesda, Maryland but the review was extended to all 'extra-mural' research supported by PHS grants and awards (studies carried out by non-governmental employees and institutions). A review by 'a committee of the investigator's institutional associates' was mandated to assure an independent determination of the rights and welfare of the individual or individuals involved, the appropriateness of the methods used to secure informed consent, and the risks and potential medical benefits of the investigation.

Since that initial step, a series of guidelines for control of bedside studies have been formulated by the US Department of Health and Human Services and by the Food and Drug Administration; similar formats have been developed in other countries.

Review committees   In these regulations, the primary responsibility for protection of research subjects is vested in institutional review committees composed of 'sufficient members with varying backgrounds to assure complete and adequate review'. Community representatives are included in many of these panels. The committees in local institutions undertake a formal evaluation of each proposed research project.

If an approved project is in need of US government financial support, it is reviewed again by a committee of experts in one of a number of specialized study sections convened by the National Institutes of Health.

GOALS OF HUMAN EXPERIMENTATION

Scientific research seems to thrive best when it is completely unrestricted and when it is not directed toward a specific practical goal. The oft quoted example of the success of a targeted research program in medicine is the crash development of a poliomyelitis vaccine, but this is outweighed by innumerable instances of unanticipated rewards from what appear to be purposeless searches for understanding about the natural world.

Freedom of inquiry in biomedical research

The issue of directed inquiry in biomedical research was examined several years ago. A review was made, by Julius H. Comroe Jr, University of California, and Robert Dripps, University of Pennsylvania, of the principal observations that led to the ten most important advances in cardiovascular and pulmonary medicine and surgery over a period of 30 years. Research efforts that had no foreseeable bearing on these problems of everyday importance in bedside medicine—the non-goal-directed investigations—paid off in terms of eventually useful discoveries almost twice as generously as other types of research and of development.

Although the 'active' observations of this after-the-fact survey provide only weak evidence of the advantages of freedom of inquiry in biomedical research, the proposition does not require a utilitarian justification. This freedom is part of a generally accepted system of values in Western societies. Isidor I. Rabi, the Nobel laureate in physics at Columbia University, put it this way, 'Science simply operates on the faith that knowledge is good and ignorance is something to overcome. You can't really vindicate this faith empirically. It *is* a faith.' Holding that conviction, he advocated an unquenchable desire for knowledge and the search for it. Others have argued conversely and with equal sincerity that there are ethical limits to discovery.

Justification for clinical studies

The controversy about limits of research is irrelevant, I believe, to the issues that arise at the threshold of clinical applications of proposals originating in the findings of pre-human studies. At the application step we must concede that *all* medical actions have consequences that extend well beyond the immediate effects seen in individual patients. As a result, we are obliged to develop arguments of policy to justify the conduct of research involving human beings. Collective justifications that point to some overall benefit for the community as a whole are the minimal requirements in the development of policy; a world view adds even more burdens to be considered. I suggest that bedside studies, unlike pre-clinical research, should be sharply goal-directed, and the goals must not be defined solely by physicians.

The fundamental distinction between the freedom to pose questions, which is essential in the search for new knowledge, and the restrictions on questions, which are necessary at the point of implementation, is not a unique demarcation made by societies. The medical profession, however, has made entreaties for a privileged position: it appeals to the humanitarian impulses of society and points to the universal desire for relief, comfort, and longevity.

> In this very serious game between the doctor and the patient, it is the latter who plays for the highest stakes; he has to bear the consequences of the medical act and is therefore interested both in the profession and in the man who practises it.
>
> J. L. Sonderegger

PRINCIPLES AND RIGHTS

Until fairly recently, doctors have exercised unrestricted discretion to intervene in the lives of their patients for the sake of medical progress. An argument of principle can be made to support this sweeping prerogative, and, in fact, a resolution adopted by the Twenty-third World Health Assembly in 1970 affirmed that the 'right to health is a fundamental human right'.

The realistic limit to assertions about a fundamental right is made clear in the line of reasoning advanced by Ronald Dworkin of New York University School of Law. The force of an argument of principle, he asserts, lies in the acceptance by a community that a person or group is entitled to some advantage or protection regardless of whether or not the community as a whole actually loses thereby. Recognition of a right commits the community to the possibility of suffering some cost in the general interest, but not necessarily a very dramatic cost.

The qualification of cost is, of course, the crucial point. A responsible government, for instance, must be ready to justify anything it does, particularly when it limits the liberty of its citizens. It is a sufficient justification, even for an act that limits liberty, that the restrictive policy is calculated to increase general utility. But there is another very important justification for limiting a right: this invokes the idea of *competing* personal rights that would be jeopardized if the right in question were not limited.

Abstract versus concrete rights   Abstract rights, like the right to health, take no account of a conflict. Concrete rights, however, reflect the impact of a competition among the rights of individual members of society. For example, we may proclaim that every infant has the right to be protected against the possibility of harmful side effects of a new treatment to prevent RLF, but this abstract right cannot be safeguarded in practice, since we can argue with equal conviction that no infant has the right to require others to undertake the unevaluated risk on his or her behalf. Thus, a strong case can be made for limiting the abstract right for a risk-free treatment by an appeal to the competing rights of those whose security will be sacrificed if the abstract right is made concrete.

Two definitions in a thesis of human rights

Policy: a kind of standard that sets out a goal to be reached, generally an improvement in some economic, political, or social feature of the community (though some goals are negative in that they stipulate that some present feature is to be protected from adverse change). Arguments of policy justify a political decision by showing that the decision advances or protects some collective goal of the community as a whole. The argument in favor of the use of public funds to conduct randomized clinical trials is an argument of policy: support will protect the populace against harmful new treatments.

Principle: a standard that is to be observed, not because it will advance or secure an economic, political, or social situation deemed desirable, but because it is a requirement of justice or fairness of some dimension of morality. Arguments of principle justify a political decision by showing that the decision respects or secures some individual or group right. The argument in favor of 'formal consent' is an argument of principle: an individual must be free to choose whether or not he or she will participate in a medical trial.

(Adapted from Dworkin)

Dworkin has proposed a human rights thesis that provides a basis for adjudicating difficult cases by confirming or denying concrete rights. But these rights, he asserts, must have two characteristics: they must be institutional rather than background rights, and they must be legal rather than some other form of institutional rights.

Institutional privileges may be found in social institutions of very different character. For example, we need some general agreement concerning the character of medicine if we are to define the prerogatives that are fixed by the distinctive rules of this institution. Needless to say, such agreement is hard to come by.

Spirit of human experimentation

In the wake of the syphilis study scandal, an ad hoc advisory panel was asked to examine the question of whether or not existing policies were adequate and effective to protect the rights of patients participating in health research supported by public funds. The panel concluded that it was the *spirit* in which an aware society undertakes to use human beings for research ends that will, ultimately, determine the protection these persons will receive.

Since the conduct of human experimentation raises important issues of social policy, greater participation is required in decision-making by representatives of non-medical professions and of the general public. But what is the 'spirit' and what is the over-arching 'social policy' that we look to for guidance?

> The people's health ... is the concern of the people themselves. They must want health. They must struggle for it and plan for it. Physicians are merely experts whose advice is sought in drawing up plans and whose cooperation is needed in carrying them out. No plan, however well designed and well intentioned, will succeed if it is imposed on the people. The war against disease and for health cannot be fought by physicians alone. It is a people's war in which the entire population must be mobilized permanently.
>
> Henry E. Sigerist

A popular war   Suppose, for the sake of argument, that we can gain general acceptance of an idea of medicine's character that sees this institution as an agency for waging a popular war. Now we can weigh some otherwise imponderable issues in realistic terms. Through this concept, we can frame questions and expect that fair-minded referees will make reasonable judgments about the rights of all concerned when new medical 'weapons' must be tested.

PATIENT RISK IN CLINICAL TRIALS

The first of the realistic issues that should be examined is the overall record of the formal approach to the testing of new treatments. Although the evidence on this point is fragmentary, there is little to support popular myth.

Outcomes in randomized clinical trials

46 Trials of Innovations in Surgery and Anesthesia

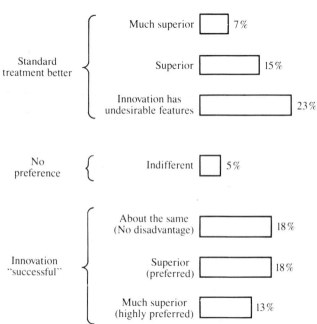

John P. Gilbert and co-workers found that innovations brought to the stage of randomized trials were 'successful' only half of the time. Results indicating that the innovations were 'highly preferred' occurred one eighth of the time.

Forfeit associated with random allotment

Ethical arguments raised when patients are to be randomly allocated to compared treatments often take one of two mutually contradictory forms.

The first contends that the routine-management group is sacrificed because they are denied the benefit of a favorable new therapy. The second argument expresses the opposite concern: patients allotted to an untested new treatment are exposed to unwarranted risk.

John P. Gilbert and his associates of Harvard University have pointed out that to a large extent, both arguments imply that the investigators know in advance which is the favorable treatment. In order to obtain some evidence on this issue, they surveyed 46 randomized clinical trials that evaluated innovations in surgery and in anesthesia. The results suggested that, on balance, new treatments showed no net gain or loss when compared with standard management. The occasional marked gains found in the survey were almost offset by clear losses, indicating that innovative treatment was usually neither better nor worse than standard treatment. In most trials, it would appear, there is little basis for selecting between compared treatments prior to the trial.

Nature and magnitude of risks

In 1976, a task force of the National Institutes of Health reported the results of a first systematic attempt to obtain an estimate of the nature and magnitude of risks for human subjects who participate in research studies. A questionnaire survey polled 538 medical investigators who had studied 39 216 patients enrolled in therapeutic trials during the previous three years. The survey analysts stressed the limitations of this weak approach to the question, but they could detect no startling dangers: there was no indication that risks in these trials were any greater than are encountered when treatments are given in other medical settings. (Most of the research-related deaths and injuries occurred in connection with the use of chemotherapy in cancer patients.)

Public attitudes

In the opening chapter, I noted that the public must be better informed about the experimental method as a risk-limiting alternative to the primitive trial and error approach that has been used in the past to evaluate innovations. I have argued throughout this volume that only critical, Galilean experiments provide the discriminatory power and efficiency we seek to safeguard the welfare of patients. (Demonstrative experiments, intended merely to illustrate 'revealed truth' and to convince others of its validity, belong in the stage presentations of faith healers.) The justification for the use of critical tests will only be accepted, Leon Eisenberg of Harvard Medical School has noted, when there is increased public awareness about the extent to which medical practice rests on custom rather than evidence, and when there is general agreement that the obligation to change this situation must be shared fairly.

Patients' attitudes   Professionals in many fields have voiced opinions about the propriety of clinical trials, but little is known about the views of those most directly affected—the patients themselves. Barrie R. Cassileth and his co-workers at the University of Pennsylvania noticed this curious gap in knowledge and sought, in 1982, to document the attitudes of current and potential patients concerning investigative treatment and participation in clinical trials. They expected to find great diversity of opinion about such an emotionally charged issue. Instead they found surprisingly uniform belief in the importance and morality of contemporary clinical trials and approval of the altruistic rationale underlying their implementation.

A questionnaire filled out anonymously by 295 respondents (104 with cancer, 84 with heart disease, and 107 'members of the public') revealed that a large majority believed patients should serve as research subjects. The responses did not differ either by subgroup or by demographic characteristics of those surveyed. Asked why they might participate in medical research, over half selected the response 'to help me get the best medical care' as their first choice. A little more than one third thought patients receiving treatment recommended by a physician receive better care; a similar proportion thought that research patients receive better treatment or that treatment is equal whether received according to trial protocol or a doctor's plan. Only one in ten stated that they would not participate in experimental studies. If the largely favorable climate of opinion found in the Philadelphia survey is at all representative, the frequent attacks on the rightfulness of clinical trials may have less popular support than is commonly believed.

Cassileth and his colleagues suggested that when those surveyed chose 'best medical care' as their major reason for participating in a clinical trial, they may have been saying, in effect, the doctor's recommendation to enroll in a trial is equivalent to that doctor's best counsel with regard to patient care. The implication of trust places a heavy ethical burden on the research physician—where it properly belongs.

RECRUITMENT OF TRIAL PARTICIPANTS

Turning now to the matter of recruiting patients to participate in clinical trials, we come to the most sensitive aspect of the issue of competing rights. The self same quandaries have been resolved in conventional warfare with the use of a draft by lottery, but there is great reluctance to consider this democratic solution to the problem of apportioning risks and benefits in medical experimentation. For example, The National Commission for the Protection of Human Subjects of Biomedical and Behavioral Research, established by an act of Congress in 1974, has advised that children who participate in research projects should be *selected* so that the burdens of participation are distributed among all segments of our society, but the recommendation is painfully silent about how this standard is to be achieved in practice.

When the American public believed it was threatened by a frightening 'enemy' in the form of paralytic poliomyelitis, hundreds of thousands of children were volunteered by their parents for participation in a randomized trial of a preventive vaccine (p 66). In this experience there was broad representation; the requirements of a democratic ideal as well as those of the rules of scientific evidence were satisfied. Such dramatic episodes are unusual. In most trials involving relatively few patients, volunteering thwarts the basic principle of random sampling which is designed to *assure* unbiased representation, and it is almost impossible to avoid gross social inequities.

Hans Jonas, the philosopher at the New School for Social Research, considered the arguments for alternatives to the volunteering approach in medical studies and rejected conscription by lot on the grounds that it was threatening and utopian. He recoiled from the idea of such a demand in a free society. I suspect he expressed the initial reaction that most of us have. But if we view formal clinical study realistically as the only fair and practical means of controlling the risks and allocating the benefits in medical development, perhaps rejection may not be so final.

Identification with the research 'cause'

The topic of patient recruitment deserves a thorough public debate. It may be argued, for example, that a requirement for the broadest possible participation in clinical studies would exert a powerful influence in ensuring the authenticity of these exercises. The question of who should be called upon to participate in clinical studies, as Jonas noted, can only be made 'right' if the 'cause' of the study is the subject's as well as the researcher's 'cause'.

> It may be accepted as a maxim that a poorly or improperly designed study involving human subjects ... is by definition unethical. Moreover, when a study is in itself scientifically invalid, all other ethical considerations become irrelevant. There is no point in obtaining 'informed consent' to perform a useless study.
>
> David Rutstein

FREELY-GIVEN INFORMED CONSENT

Another thorny matter that must be faced in human experimentation revolves around the concept of consent. How can we fulfill the letter and spirit of the International Code of Ethics which specifies that each potential subject must be adequately informed and that he or she should grant freely-given consent? The stipulation that consent be obtained in writing presents no difficulties, but it is virtually impossible to comply fully with the *intent* of the rule..

It has been pointed out that the very justification for a randomized trial is that there is insufficient information to permit a rational informed choice. Moreover, an explanation of the technical issues and an offer of choice of whether or not to enroll, give little assurance of compliance with the spirit of the ethics code. The quality of consent is often influenced by the social relationship of the principals; this quality is simply not the same when there is a wide social gap between doctor and patient as it is when they are more nearly social equals. It also cannot be denied that self-interest can make the research physician very persuasive.

Acquiescence of surrogates

Communal consent   Carl E. Taylor of Johns Hopkins University has called attention to complications that arise when clinical trials are conducted in countries where health decisions are typically made by the family and the community. When most decisions about treatment are communal, is it only a facade, he asks, to insist on individual consent? The international guidelines endorsed in 1981 recognized the problem. When individual members of a rural community in developing countries do not have the necessary awareness of the implications of participation in an experiment, the guidelines advise that the decision whether or not to participate should be elicited through the intermediary of a trusted community leader. The intermediary should make it clear that any eligible person is free to abstain or withdraw at any time.

Obsession with individual decision making in developed countries may obscure the general importance of distinguishing between situations that require personal consent and those which require community approval. The latter may be appropriate when a particular health measure has been sufficiently tested to be ready for a mass trial in a public health program.

'Permission' of guardians   The concept of acquiescence when children and others not competent to understand the issues are involved in experimental trials has been considered at great length by many individuals and official groups. A review was undertaken by the President's National Commission which advised that the word 'consent' in this context be abandoned. The advisory group suggested that the 'permission' of parents or guardians be solicited to distinguish what a person may do autonomously (consent) from what one may do on behalf of another (grant permission). There is general agreement that, to the extent feasible, older children should be given the opportunity to make their own decisions with the additional permission of the parent or other legal guardian.

An additional suggestion made by the commission concerned the active involvement of traditional protectors. For example, it advised that small children should participate in certain investigations only if their parents or guardians agree to be present during some or all of the conduct of the research. In general, the parents should be sufficiently involved in the research to understand its effects on their children and be able to intervene, if necessary.

Informed surveillance I have proposed a plan for clinical trials which I have termed 'informed surveillance'. The objective is to enlist the active participation of personal physicians. In this format the investigator is charged with the responsibilities of informing the personal physician of a prospective enrollee about the details of the study protocol and answering questions that arise at all stages of the study. The personal physician, who must not be the investigator under this division of responsibilities, is charged with the task of *attempting* to inform the patient or guardian about the trial and requesting written permission in which the patient confirms only that he or she has *no objections* to proceeding.

This oblique form of assent, I have argued, makes no assumption that the patient *fully* understands the explanation provided. The more completely informed personal physician—as in day-to-day practice—acts as the intermediary who defends the rights and personal welfare of his or her patient. Moreover, both the patient and the personal physician retain veto options that may be exercised at any stage of the investigation. They should not be made to feel any obligation to adhere to the agreement made at the time of enrollment in a clinical trial; 'second thoughts' should be respected without coercion.

Discretionary informing

Conscientious doctors are in the habit of using discretion when they discuss illness and treatment with individual patients. In weighing the consequences of complete candor they usually wait for a clue from patients, some of whom make it clear that they wish to know every detail; others indicate they wish to be told very little when they say, 'I leave everything up to you, Doctor.' Arguments have been made that this usual practice of discretionary informing should be considered as an alternative to the rigid informed consent procedure in many clinical trials. The modification runs counter to the demand that all trial participants must be fully informed, but it is quite realistic. The discretionary approach received indirect support in a survey conducted by R.J. Simes and M.H.N. Tattersall of the University of Sydney; most of the patients surveyed believed that they alone should decide the extent of disclosure in randomized trials. Cassileth has shown that patients often avoid reading consent agreements which they have signed because they regard the documents as legalistic, undesirable intrusions into the trust relationship with their doctors.

A balance sometimes needs to be struck between the fear that patients' rights will be violated if they are not fully informed and the fact that some patients will be made to suffer undue anxiety as the result of full disclosure. There is a special need for compromise when consent is obtained for treatment of disorders in patients who have no symptoms and regard themselves as completely well.

Disavowals in clinical trials

Human experimentation faces practical hindrances which frustrate investigators who chafe at the inefficiency of clinical trials. A basic impediment is erected by a free society's commitment to the principle of self-direction or autonomy, according to which an individual reaches practical decisions as the result of independent and rational reflection. Patients have the right of informed *dissent*. This source of 'inefficiency' is, I believe, an essential restraint that must not be set aside.

Uncooperative participants   If the veto options of enrolled patients are exercised so frequently that a trial is 'ruined', the significance of this turn of events should not be overlooked. From a community oriented perspective, the rates of non-compliance and defection by patients (and by personal physicians in an informed surveillance plan) are basic pieces of information.

Since a major warrant for *human* experiments lies in the potential for projecting results to the community at large, bedside trials should be designed to generate useful information bearing on this fundamental objective. If patients and personal physicians are unable to identify with the goals of the trial and do not perceive themselves as active participants, there is little reason to expect that an outcome of interest to the investigator will be of any public interest. It makes no sense to develop potent weapons to fight an unpopular war.

Alienation of practitioners and communities   As I proposed above, special efforts should be made to enlist the aid and to stimulate the interest of practicing physicians in formal clinical trials, for it is the practitioner who must translate the results of trials into everyday usage. The disturbing effect when personal physicians feel alienated from research efforts has been documented. Chalmers examined the extent to which the practice of medicine is a reflection of controlled clinical trials and found a number of examples in which there was a clear-cut dichotomy between the 'usual practice of the community' and the scientific data. Physicians seemed to be paying no attention to the results of carefully designed studies.

Community acceptance of research results also may founder when there is little public representation in the planning of large-scale trials. The problem is seen most clearly when field trials conducted in developing countries are set up at the request of research workers in the developed world.

Obligation to freely consenting participants

What is the responsibility of the community to the recruits in medical studies? Schemes for compensating persons injured by immunizations, which are obligatory or recommended by health authorities, currently exist in a number of countries. An international conference on the role of the individual and the community in the development of biologicals (such as vaccines, toxoids, and antisera) has advised that governments enlarge the concept of support of medical research to include reparation for the inevitable casualties that occur. There is growing awareness of the need to assume this public obligation. It is inescapable that the benefits of well designed research are shared by society as a whole, whereas the risks are endured by the few who participate as experimental subjects.

No-fault reparation A system of obtaining payment from a centrally administered fund without proving fault has much to commend it as a satisfactory way of compensating for injuries received in the course of medical research. Under this arrangement, researchers and participants do not find themselves in the position of adversaries, and researchers may assist an injured recruit in assembling evidence for the claim. No-fault compensation schemes are already operating in at least three countries—Sweden, New Zealand, and the Federal Republic of Germany.

PUBLIC CHARACTER OF SCIENTIFIC MEDICINE

Medicine's ancient roots have left a lasting impression on the character of this healing art. Its early history is closely connected with the history of religion and this association goes a long way in explaining physicians' strange claims of righteousness when it comes to making value judgments and taking actions that affect the lives of others. For example, unbridled human experiments designed to 'save lives' are rationalized by an 'ends justify the means' principle which has its origin in religious doctrine. A seventeenth century Jesuit moralist, Busenbaum, defended the proposition *cum finis est lictus, etiam media sunt licita* (if the end is lawful, the means

---

Human institutions are so imperfect by their nature that in order to destroy them it is almost always enough to extend their underlying ideas to the extreme.

Alexis de Tocqueville

are also lawful). This argument has since been renounced by Jesuits, but it has tended to linger on in medicine.

Role of medical knowledge in human affairs

What is the role of professional knowledge and action in human affairs? Sociologist Eliot Freidson of New York University has suggested that medicine offers the best test of the general question of whether the ends of established professions are so humanitarian that experts may be given the autonomy to lead all of society to them. Ideally, in medicine, actions are based on reliable objective evidence, and what the profession deems to be good, the public, on the surface, regards as good. However, there lies at the bottom of medicine's applied efforts a moral rather than an objective judgment. Further, the professionally defined 'good' is asserted to be worth the price the patient is asked to pay in relinquishing his independence. But unless the moral foundation of medicine is identical to that of the community, it will serve not the community but itself.

Limits of professional dominance   Freidson examined the limits of professional authority and concluded that the professions, no matter how beneficent their intent, have neither the special qualifications nor the moral right to make choices for the individual or for society.

> What a man calls moral judgment is merely his desire to generalize, and so make available for others, those values he has come to choose.
>
> C. Wright Mills

Physicians often make the assumption that medical practice, especially when it is based on sound evidence, is a pure, moral, acultural activity. I believe that it is this issue—the conflict between value judgments of doctors and patients and their families—that is at the heart of the profession's well-founded fear that enlargement of the public role in all matters relating to human investigation will slow the rate of technical development. The medical profession is puzzled by a strange paradox: as medicine becomes more effective it receives more public criticism. I do not find this at all surprising and it is certainly not anti-scientific; sharp criticism is part and parcel of the scientific method.

Scientific medicine is not seen as having the property of closure or finality—a fixed body of undoubted knowledge and a limited set of unquestioned concepts. It is seen, rather, as an evolving, open-ended search and the uncertainties are very much the concern of everybody.

Social aspect of the scientific method

As medicine leaves religion and mysticism behind, abandons its secretive and authoritarian past, and becomes more scientific, it will move in the direction of openness. This means, I suggest, that it will become more responsive to human need than heretofore. What must be understood is that the scientific method has a public character. It flourishes only when there is free criticism that is not deterred by authorities.

Popper has emphasized this aspect of scientific objectivity: theories are expressed in a form that can be tested by anyone who has taken the time to learn the technique of understanding and evaluating scientific hypotheses.

The Robinson Crusoe parable In order to illustrate the social aspect of the scientific method, Popper asks us to suppose that Robinson Crusoe succeeded in building physical and chemical laboratories, an astronomical observatory, and so forth, during the period of isolation from the rest of the world on his remote island. Further, suppose that he wrote many papers, based on observation and experiment. We are also to assume that he succeeded in describing scientific systems that coincided with the results then currently accepted by mainland scientists.

Considering the character of Crusonian science, we may be inclined to regard it as authentic because the islander used the painstaking methodology of the natural sciences. But, Popper reminds us, a vital element of the scientific method is missing. There was nobody but himself to check his results, nobody but himself to correct those prejudices that are the unavoidable consequences of his unique mental history, nobody to help him get rid of that strange blindness concerning the inherent possibilities of his own results that is a consequence of the fact that most of them were reached through comparatively irrelevant approaches. Consequently, the fact that Crusoe arrived at conventional results, without the carping of critics, is nearly as accidental and miraculous as it would be if they were conjured by a clairvoyant.

Concerning Crusoe's papers, it is only in attempts to explain his work to somebody who has not done it that he can acquire the discipline of clear reasoned communication, which is also part of the scientific method. Thus, it may be said that what we call 'scientific objectivity' is not the product of the individual investigator's impartiality but a summation of the social or public character of the scientific method.

Give me a good fruitful error anytime, full of seeds bursting with its own corrections. You can keep the sterile truth for yourself.

The Practical Cogitator

It is openness to criticism rather than philosophical arguments, I submit, that constitutes the most substantial hope that scientific medicine will remain humane and responsive to human need. Even a society made wary of science, because of misapplication of technical developments, must know that the underlying logical machinery of the scientific method is in the public interest.

Science, Popper pointed out, is one of the very few human activities in which errors are systematically criticized and fairly often, in time, corrected.

Appendix A
The story of retrolental fibroplasia

A 'NEW' DISEASE

Retrolental fibroplasia (literally, fibrous tissue behind the lens of the eye) was 'discovered' in February 1941 by two Boston physicians—pediatrician Stewart H. Clifford and ophthalmologist Paul A. Chandler. They examined a three-month-old girl and found what appeared to be dense white membranes filling the pupils of her eyes; the abnormalities were unlike anything they had ever seen before. This blind baby and four additional RLF-affected children were reported the following year in a preliminary note by Boston ophthalmologist, Theodore L. Terry. He found that all five of the patients had been born prematurely. 'In view of these findings,' he wrote prophetically, 'perhaps this complication should be expected in a certain percentage of premature infants. If so, some new factors have arisen in extreme prematurity to produce such a condition.'

Rising frequency

The prediction was fulfilled; following the initial report, Terry examined well over a hundred children with the strange type of infant blindness by the time of his death in 1946. Search of past records revealed that the unusual condition had been noted sporadically (under a variety of obscure labels) for more than 30 years, but there was little question that it was now occurring as a fairly common complication of extreme prematurity (the condition was less frequent in relatively mature babies and rare in full-term infants). Surveys conducted in cities throughout the world confirmed a suspicion that the complication seemed to occur most frequently in infants reared in premature centers with the most highly organized and advanced programs for care.

Descriptive studies

During the first years of study, affected babies were examined when they were several months old. It was assumed that the disorder had developed before or, at the latest, immediately after birth. Retrospective studies focused on associations with complications of pregnancy and delivery, and with treatments given to m⁄ thers or to their offspring immediately after premature birth.

Prospective observations

Understanding was improved after the results of a prospective investigation were reported. William and Ella Owens, a husband and wife team of ophthalmologists at Johns Hopkins University, examined more than 200 prematurely born infants in a hospital nursery; all had normal eyes. Half of these babies were examined at regular intervals; 4 per cent developed RLF. They described a progressive development of proliferative blood vessel changes (manifested by dilation and tortuosity of retinal arteries and veins seen in the interior of the eye with an ophthalmoscope) beginning at age $2\frac{1}{2}$–$3\frac{1}{2}$ months in the afflicted babies. Soon there were retinal hemorrhages, the retinal layer of the eye became elevated and grayish masses of detaching retinal tissue billowed forward in the chamber of the eye and formed an opaque scar-like cast behind the lens. At this stage of the abnormal process (at 4–6 months of age), the pupil of the eye appeared white even to an untrained observer. Both eyes were usually involved and, not infrequently, the severity of the scarring changes was unequal. It was now clear that the disorder usually began well after delivery, and focus of interest shifted to postnatal events and treatments.

The frequency of occurrence of RLF, first in the United States and later in other developed countries, rose sharply at the end of the 1940s. It quickly became the leading form of blindness in infants, but peculiar geographic and temporal differences in incidence were reported.

Circumstantial associations

An attempt to seek an explanation for the alarming new epidemic was undertaken in 1949. The co-occurrences of RLF and 47 factors relating to mothers and children (298 normal and 53 RLF-afflicted children) delivered in Boston during the years 1938–48 were examined. A number of associations were discovered. The most interesting were those related to treatments: the rise in incidence paralleled the use of medicinal iron, water-miscible vitamins, and supplemental oxygen. The investigators found, however, that the correlation 'was less striking for oxygen than for ... vitamin preparations and for iron' (p 17). Numerous other associations were described in a flood of anecdotal reports published in the late 1940s and early 1950s.

EARLY COMPARATIVE TRIALS

Vitamin E

The results of the Boston survey led to a suggestion that the eye condition might be related to vitamin E deficiency (marginal body stores of this substance at birth aggravated by the use of water-miscible vitamins that increased the requirement for vitamin E, and by a destructive effect of iron salts on the E substance—alpha tocopherol). The hypothesis was tested in a quasi-experimental trial for a period of 10 months (alternate infants admitted to a premature nursery in Baltimore during 1949 received either synthetic vitamin E or no treatment). The early trend of difference in the two groups (no RLF among 11 treated infants, 5 developed the condition in the control group of 15 babies) was sufficient to impress advisers who were keeping an eye on the study; they persuaded the researchers to abandon the controlled trial. Subsequently all infants received vitamin E treatment, and, as word of the Baltimore experience spread, the preventive treatment was started in many hospitals throughout the world. These experiences showed no impressive protective effect of tocopherol treatment; after a few years, all interest in this approach faded away.

ACTH

Following the vitamin E disappointment, numerous other treatments were tried. One of the most promising of these was the use of a powerful agent ACTH (adrenocorticotropic hormone), to inhibit the wild proliferation of retinal blood vessels seen on examination of the eye in the early stages of RLF. At a New York Hospital, 31 infants with vascular changes were treated with ACTH; 25 experienced a regression of the abnormalities and they were left with completely normal eyes. By contrast, 7 babies at a nearby hospital had not been treated when they showed early signs of the affliction; 6 of the 7 went on to become totally blind.

ACTH seemed to be the cure for the disease. But further studies quickly dashed this hope. A formal randomized clinical trial of the new treatment—ACTH compared with untreated controls *in the same hospital*—indicated that the outlook was better for babies who were untreated. The potent therapy had been without appreciable effect on what is ordinarily a benign course (later studies demonstrated that early changes of RLF usually subside spontaneously), and the investigators were disturbed to find that ACTH-treated infants appeared to have a higher risk of fatal infections.

SUPPLEMENTAL OXYGEN

First associations

In 1951—a full decade after the 'discovery' of the affliction—oxygen enriched incubators were implicated by association. Expensive, gas-tight American incubators had been introduced in Britain when the newly inaugurated National Health Service provided the funds to pay for them. RLF began to appear shortly thereafter. Mary Crosse, a Birmingham pediatrician, wondered aloud whether or not the disease might be linked to the new equipment. An Australian doctor, Kate Campbell, set out to confirm Crosse's idea by tallying the outcomes in infants who had been treated with different oxygen regimens in three Melbourne hospitals. Her observations connected the eye disease to liberal use of supplemental oxygen (p 18).

Conflicting observations

When other investigators tried to confirm Campbell's circumstantial evidence, the results were confusing. A survey in Oxford partially supported the oxygen hypothesis, however, a hospital in New Orleans found no RLF among oxygen-exposed babies. A Paris group observed that infants treated with continuous high concentrations of oxygen were no more likely to develop blindness than others who received the medicinal gas only sparingly. And the findings of Thaddeus Szewczyk, an ophthalmologist in East St Louis, seemed to contradict the 'oxygen is dangerous' theory completely. Szewczyk believed that RLF developed when babies were removed from high concentrations of oxygen too quickly. When the early signs of blood vessel abnormality were observed in 19 infants, they were returned to high oxygen environments; all improved and their eyes became normal after four days.

A quasi-experimental trial

Two young physicians, ophthalmology house officer Arnall Patz and pediatrician Leroy Hoeck, attempted to conduct a controlled clinical trial of oxygen treatment in a Washington D.C. hospital. Seventy-six small premature infants were assigned in alternate order to liberal oxygen or to restricted oxygen regimens. The results of this trial, published in 1952, seemed to indict continuous oxygen treatment. But the investigators and their critics had a number of unresolved doubts about the trial: compliance with the prescribed treatments was questionable (p 107), the potential bias introduced by non-random assignments could not be evaluated, 11 infants were withdrawn or dropped out, and fears about the matter of safety of oxygen restriction (risk of death and of brain damage) could not be allayed by the small experience.

Animal evidence

Research with experimental animals was also frustrating. In the early 1950s, British ophthalmologist Norman Ashton found that exposure to oxygen in high concentrations caused changes in the eyes of newborn kittens that exactly mimicked the early stages of the human disease; the blood vessels in the retina first constricted, the immature vascular network then withered, and this was followed by wild proliferation of vascular tissue when the kittens were removed from oxygen. These experiments strongly supported a role of supplemental oxygen in the genesis of RLF, except for one crucial limitation. The animals, unlike human infants with the disease, never became blind. Thus, doubts persisted concerning the prime cause of blinding complications in babies.

A national trial

By early 1953, it became obvious that the confused picture concerning the associations between care-taking practices and outcomes (RLF, death, and brain damage) would only be clarified by means of a large scale critical experiment using a newly devised investigative plan—the randomized clinical trial. It was hoped that this would lead to the prevention of a disease that had, by this time, blinded about 10 000 infants throughout the world (approximately 7000 of the victims were born in the United States).

A meeting was convened in early 1953 by the US Public Health Service; most of the American pediatricians and ophthalmologists who had been studying the epidemic were invited. Although the majority felt that a controlled trial must be undertaken immediately, a minority felt that excess oxygen had already been demonstrated to be the cause of RLF and that it was immoral to expose infants to the high oxygen treatment regimen that had been used for years in the routine management of small babies. A still smaller group believed that treatment with high oxygen concentrations was absolutely necessary to ensure intact survival; they argued that the proposed new approach of oxygen curtailment was unethical. The great divergence of opinion showed, as much as anything, that a definitive, well controlled trial was essential to settle the controversial issues. It was finally agreed that 18 hospitals throughout the US would join in a cooperative effort to compare the effects of two contrasting regimens of oxygen administration.

A fixed time period of one year was chosen by the planners (it was estimated that 750 infants would be available for study during this interval). A complex design for random allocation to treatments was chosen: for three months two thirds of the enrolled infants were to be managed according to the new curtailed-oxygen policy, while one third were to receive routine treatment of continuous high concentrations of the gas. Mortality rates were to be closely monitored during this initial phase of the trial; if no dangers of oxygen restriction were detected, all enrolled babies would be managed under the curtailed-oxygen regimen for the remaining nine months of the trial. In view of the many disappointments and false hopes of the past, all participants in the trial agreed that no results should be released until the carefully planned exercise was completed and all the accumulated data were analyzed. The complicated clinical trial began on 1 July 1953.

'Under 40 per cent is safe'

In May 1954 a publication appeared reporting the results of a single-hospital randomized clinical trial comparing the effects of high versus low oxygen therapy (under 40 per cent concentration) among 85 premature infants. Mortality in the low-oxygen group was greater than among those who were assigned to liberal oxygen, but the difference was attributed to chance (p 122). No instances of scarring RLF were observed among 28 survivors in low oxygen; 8 examples were found among 36 surviving babies treated with high oxygen. The authors concluded that a policy of oxygen restriction was not harmful and that RLF was entirely preventable if oxygen (kept below 40 per cent) was administered only when necessary. Many observers, noting the small number of infants in the study, chose to await the results of the national trial before altering the methods of care that might increase mortality or brain damage. But the suspense and concerns grew as the final months of the large study dragged on.

Epidemic conquered

In September 1954 (after the eyes of the last enrollees in June were followed for three months) the results of the collaborative effort were announced. No appreciable increase in mortality had been observed under restricted oxygen, but there appeared to be a striking reduction in scarring RLF: 23 per cent of 53 babies who had received standard high concentrations of oxygen (above 50 per cent for 28 days) were affected; 7 per cent of 533 infants in the curtailed group (only as indicated and under 50 per cent oxygen concentration) developed the permanent lesions of the eye disorder. Physicians were warned that supplemental oxygen should no longer be administered on a routine basis. It was advised that the gas should be administered only when absolutely necessary and that both the duration of treatment and concentration of oxygen should be kept to a minimum.

The battle to eliminate the twelve-year scourge of premature infants seemed to be won at last—the incidence of RLF dropped precipitously around the world as restricted-oxygen policy was widely adopted. In the flush of success it was forgotten that the original plans called for monitoring the long-term neurologic status of the large number of infants enrolled in the unique US study. Follow-up studies of these children were never carried out.

A PYRRHIC VICTORY

As it turned out, the victory over RLF was not as glorious as first thought, but it took years to piece together what may have happened. Epidemiologic evidence began to suggest that RLF had virtually disappeared because the infants at highest risk were dying in the first hours of life. (This fact lay buried in summaries of mortality rates which were not analyzed by age at death and by birthweight.) The frequency of the most common fatal lung disorder in the smallest premature infants (hyaline membrane disease) and overall first-day mortality in the most immature babies both increased as RLF fell. Equally disturbing was an apparent increase in the number of premature infants who developed a form of cerebral palsy (spastic diplegia) during the years after 1954 when the policy of oxygen restriction was in effect. A British follow-up study of children who had been born prematurely, reported in 1962 by Alison D. McDonald, then of Guy's Hospital Medical School, found a correlation between spastic diplegia and postnatal breathing disorders, and an inverse relationship between the rate of brain damage and duration of oxygen treatment.

Over-interpretation of evidence

The findings came as a shock since the national cooperative study and single-hospital trials had seemed to provide clear answers about the relationship between oxygen treatment and RLF. In retrospect, it was realized that many of the interpretations had been unwarranted. The single-hospital trials were too small to test the mortality question vigorously and the cooperative trial enrolled infants too late— they were enlisted at age two days. Since the first 48 hours of life is the period of highest mortality risk (a full 45 per cent of premature infants admitted to the 18 collaborating hospitals died before they were old enough to be enrolled), the 'curtailment of oxygen is safe' question had not been put to a critical test in the national study. The suspicion slowly grew that oxygen was being restricted too stringently, particularly in the crucial first two days of life. But the agonizing question was never put to a formal test.

The confusing situation in the 1960s was further complicated by the widely broadcast claim that RLF would not occur if oxygen concentration was kept under 40 per cent (based on extrapolation of results in the small single-hospital trial reported in May 1954). Again, the possibilities of a critical threshold of oxygen concentration, a critical duration of exposure, or some combination measure of oxygen dosage were never tested by means of formal experiment. Moreover, questions about the exact role of supplemental oxygen began to surface when it was found that RLF in premature infants who were *never* exposed to the gas was not rare; some examples were discovered in stillborn infants (who had never been exposed to 21 per cent oxygen in ordinary room air).

DETERMINATIVE ERA OF OXYGEN TREATMENT

In the late 1960s, physicians cautiously began to administer oxygen more liberally than in the post-1954 years of strict curtailment. A new technical development—measurement of oxygen tension in minute samples of arterial blood—made it possible to monitor the oxygen status of treated babies. It was hoped that this new determinative approach would now make it possible to administer oxygen so precisely that the twin dangers of too little and too much of the gaseous substance could be avoided. This was a very reasonable expectation; unfortunately, the exact definition of safe limits of arterial oxygen were unknown and it was considered unethical to carry out an experimental trial to determine this vital information. (Studies in experimental animals were not applicable because other species did not exhibit scarring lesions and blindness when exposed to oxygen.)

The relatively weak investigative approaches of analytic surveys and, in one instance, a collaborative observational study, failed to provide clear-cut answers to the perplexing questions that plagued treating physicians. (For example, the observational study found no association between arterial oxygen and RLF risk; circumstantial evidence that linked duration of oxygen treatment and risk was uninterpretable because oxygen was administered to infants according to physician prescription, that is, on an as-needed basis.)

Resurgence of RLF

During the 1970s, life-support techniques were perfected to the point that the survival rate of very small premature infants increased sharply. With this rise it slowly became evident that RLF increased apace. Despite improved techniques of monitoring the oxygen status of these very small infants—by continuous measurement using sensors applied to the skin—the estimated number of RLF-afflicted babies seen each year began to approach pre-1954 levels.

As the 1980s began, the oxygen hypothesis was badly shaken. There was reason to think that oxygen exposure played a role in the development of retinal blood vessel changes, but it was obvious that understanding about the complex mechanisms responsible for producing the irreversible complication of blindness after premature birth was far from complete.

Appendix B
Checklist for randomized clinical trial design

1 Selection description—clear portrayal of patients studied
2 Reject log—record of eligible population *not* accepted for the trial
3 Withdrawals—dropouts listed by diagnosis, treatment, and reason for withdrawal
4 Therapeutic regimens defined—includes timing, amount of daily therapies and all (additional) allowable therapies
5 Control regimen—placebo appearance and taste
6 Masking procedures
   a Randomization masking—unpredictability of upcoming treatment assignment
   b Masking of patients—therapy unidentified
   c Masking of physicians—therapy unidentified
   d Masking of physicians and patients—ongoing results of the trial are hidden
7 Testing procedures
   a Sizing the study—prior estimate of number of patients required (Δ, and risk levels α and β)
   b Distribution of pretreatment variables—known prognostic features by treatment category
   c Evaluation of masking—physicians and patients queried at the end of the study
   d Compliance—objective methods of verifying conforming behavior of patients and physicians
   e Biological equivalent—attempt to measure therapeutic agent in its active form (after absorption or injection)
8 Statistical analysis
   a Statistical significance of end points—both test statistic and observed probability stated
   b β estimate—discussion of Type II error
   c Statistical inference—confidence limits, lifetable or time-series analysis, regression analyses or correlations
9 Handling of withdrawals—convention adopted for withdrawals
10 Side effects—report and discuss side effects of therapies
11 Retrospective analyses—post hoc analysis of results in sub-groups with due caution concerning conclusion
12 Masking of statistician—presentation of data to analyst in coded form.

13 Problem of multiple looks—consider influence of multiple analyses of accumulating data
14 Supplementary data
    a Dates of starting and stopping accessions
    b Results of pre-randomization data analysis—evaluation of baseline com-
parability of study groups
    c Tabulation of events employed as end-points for each treatment
    d Timing of events—event times (e.g. outcomes, withdrawals) given to permit
construction of a plot of outcome against time
(Compiled by Chalmers and co-workers)

Further reading
(Alphabetic order by title)

Assessing the Social Impacts of Medical Technologies.
  H. David Banta & Joshua R. Sanes. *J. Community Health* (1978) **3**, 245–58
  A general discussion of the principles for assessing
  indirect effects of new medical techniques on
  individuals or on social systems.
Causal Thinking in the Health Sciences. Mervyn Susser.
  Oxford Univ. Press, 1973
  A well written book that provides working concepts with which to interpret
  environmental influences on health.
Clinical Epidemiology. Alvan R. Feinstein, W.B. Saunders Co, 1985
  An excellent (detailed) discussion of the structure of clinical investigative methods,
  including the 'architecture' of randomized clinical trials.
Clinical Trials. Daniel Schwartz, Robert Flamant & Joseph Lellouch (transl. M.J.R.
  Healy). Academic Press. 1980
  A practical guide for human experimentation in which the important distinction
  between 'explanatory' and 'pragmatic' approaches is made explicit.
Conjectures and Refutations: The Growth of Scientific Knowledge. Karl R. Popper.
  Basic Books, 1962
  A collection of highly readable essays in which Popper develops his thesis that
  our knowledge grows through correcting our mistakes.
Controlled Clinical Trials. Official Journal of the Society for Clinical Trials. Pub-
  lished quarterly by Elsevier North Holland, Inc.
  An international journal that publishes articles dealing with the design, methods,
  and operational aspects of prospective studies with emphasis on controlled clinical
  trials.
Design and Analysis of Randomized Clinical Trials Requiring Prolonged Observation of Each Patient. Richard Peto *et al. B. J. Cancer* (1976) **34**, 585–612, and
  (1977) **35**, 1–39
  An exceptionally clear set of instructions and examples for design and analysis of
  long term clinical trials; intended for readers without statistical expertise.
Ethics and Regulation of Clinical Research. Robert J. Levine. Urban & Schwarzen-
  berg, 1981
  A thorough survey of the ethical and legal duties of clinical investigators, including an explication of the President's Commission ... 1981 biennial report on the
  protection of human subjects.

The Historical Development of Clinical Therapeutic Trials. J.P. Bull. *J. Chronic Diseases* (1959) **10,** 218–48

An interesting review of methods of therapeutic investigation from antiquity (procedures described in the Edwin Smith papyrus, *ca* 1600 BC) to the period just preceding the modern randomized controlled clinical trial (1949–51).

How to Read Clinical Journals ... [a series]. David L. Sackett. *J. Can. Med. Assoc.* (1981) **124,** 555–8, 703–10, 869–72, 985–90, and 1156–62

An invaluable set of guidelines for approaching the expanding volume of published medical reports. The timely recommendations are designed to assist readers who must separate the 'wheat from the chaff' in claims of innovation in diagnosis, prognosis, and therapy.

Induction and Intuition in Scientific Thought. Peter B. Medawar. American Philosophical Society, 1969

A reflective discussion of the shift from Baconian induction to critical experimentation in modern science.

An Introduction to the Study of Experimental Medicine. Claude Bernard (Transl. H.C. Greene). Henry Schuman, Inc., 1949

A translation of the classic treatise published in 1865 which describes the successive steps of scientific analysis and Claude Bernard's interpretation of the way in which the mind of a scientist goes to work on a problem.

The Logic of Chance. John Venn. Chelsea Publishing Co., 1962

(This 'Fourth Edition' is an unaltered reprint of the third edition published in 1888.)

A classic exposition of the theory of probability; the physical foundations and logical superstructure of the theory are discussed with unusual charm and clarity.

The Logic of Medicine. Edmond A. Murphy. Johns Hopkins Univ. Press, 1976

An excellent book that sets out in an engaging manner to cultivate an 'alert common sense' concerning the rules of evidence in medicine.

'A Logical Analysis of Medicine'. W.I. Card & I.J. Good in *A Companion to Medical Studies.* R. Passmore & J.S. Robson (Eds.). Blackwell Scientific Publications, 1974 Chapter 60 in this work presents a lucid discussion of the application of decision theory to medicine.

The Profession of Medicine. Eliot Freidson. Dodd, Mead & Co., 1972

A fascinating sociological analysis of the profession of medicine: a prime example of the sociology of applied knowledge.

Radicals and Squares. Richard B. Darlington. Logan Hill Press, 1975

An introduction to statistics written in a relaxed narrative style, supplemented with very useful chapter summaries and flow-charts.

Retrolental Fibroplasia: A Modern Parable. W.A. Silverman. Grune & Stratton, 1980

An interpretive review of the retrolental fibroplasia 'epidemic' and its implications.

Taking Rights Seriously. Ronald Dworkin. Harvard Univ. Press, 1977

A well argued definition and defense of a liberal theory of law.

Note that the National Perinatal Epidemiology Unit is a fertile information resource with considerable experience in the organization and management of multicenter randomized trials. The Unit is located in Radcliffe Infirmary, Oxford OX2 6HE, England.

The Clinical Trials Centre is available to help and advise doctors about to embark on large prospective randomized trials in the treatment of cancer. The Centre is located in Rayne Institute, King's College Hospital Medical School, London SE5 8RX, England.

Acknowledgments and citations

I am grateful to Richard L. Day for his advice after reading an early draft of this book. Iain Chalmers, Director of Britain's National Perinatal Epidemiology Unit, read the penultimate draft and made many valuable suggestions. It is a pleasure to acknowledge his wise counsel and to thank him for his many kind acts. My wife's contributions to this volume are substantial and I cannot thank her enough for her help and sensible suggestions.

I am very much indebted to the many authors whose evidence and opinions I have cited in this book. They are identified by name in the text or in legends for tables and graphs. The published source of the citations are given below in the order in which they occur in each chapter. I gratefully acknowledge the permission of copyright holders to use their material. In some cases permission has been impossible to obtain due to lack of available information as to the true copyright holder, despite every reasonable effort.

PREFACE

Burnet's comments are in *Lancet* (1953) **i,** 103–8.

For Susser's microscope analogy see Further Reading: *Causal Thinking ...*

Braunwald's comment is in *Hospital Practice* (1971) **6,** 910.

Critical rationalism is discussed by Popper, see Further Reading: *Conjectures ...*

The toy set analogy is in Goffman's *Relations in Public* (1971), Basic Books.

CHAPTER 1

Part of this chapter was included in the Apgar Award Lecture published in *Perspectives in Biology and Medicine* (1981) **24,** 339–51.

For Webster's discussion of Bacon's thesis see *The Great Instauration: Science, Medicine and Reform 1626-60* (1976), Holmes and Meier.

The contrast between Bacon's experiments and those of Galileo is made clear by Medawar, see Further Reading: *Induction and ...*

For Bernard's comments see Further Reading: *An Introduction ...*

Lind's experiment is described in *A Treatise of the Scurvey* (1953 reprint of the 1753 publication), Edinburgh Univ. Press.

Galbraith's aphorism is in *The New Industrial State* (1971), Houghton and Mifflin.

The unwitting experiment data is in *Snow on Cholera* (1936 reprint of John Snow's 1855 treatise), Commonwealth Fund.

Fisher's discussion is in *J. Min. Agriculture* (1926) **33**, 503–13.

The roles of Karl Pearson and others are discussed by Mainland in *Clin. Pharm. Therap.* (1960) **1**, 411–22 and (1963) **4**, 580–6.

The tuberculosis treatment trial is discussed in Hill's *Statistical Methods in Clinical and Preventive Medicine* (1962), Oxford Univ. Press.

The choice between studies is adapted from Susser; see Further Reading: *Causal Thinking . . .*

Fredrickson's comment is in *Bull. N.Y. Acad. Med.* (1968) **44**, 985–93.

CHAPTER 2

Postman's story is in *Crazy Talk, Stupid Talk* (1976), Delacorte.

For Popper's argument see Further Reading: *Conjectures . . .*

For Bernard's levels of observation see Further Reading: *An Introduction . . .*

The line graph of 'passive' association in the Boston survey is redrawn (with permission) from Kinsey and Zacharias in *J. Am. Med. Assoc.* (1949) **139**, 572–8.

Rarity, interest, and surprise are discussed by Weaver in *The Scientific Monthly* (1949) **67**, 390–2.

Data in the Melbourne table (copyright 1951 M.J.A.) are Campbell's in *Med. J. Aust.* (1951) **2**, 48–50.

The sailor's misunderstanding is quoted by Levinson in *The Science of Chance* (1939), Rinehart.

Selvin and Stuart's data-dredging metaphors are in *The American Statistician* (1966) **20**, 20–3.

Data in the 'hunting accident' table are from Allen and others in *N. Eng. J. Med.* (1949) **241**, 799–806.

Galton's contribution is described by Pearson in *Life and Letters of Francis Galton* (1934), Cambridge Univ. Press.

Causal relationships are discussed by Susser, see Further Reading: *Causal Thinking . . .*

The London Bill of Mortality is from David's *Games, Gods and Gambling* (1962), Charles Griffen and Co.; Petty's quotation is from Greenwood in *Biometrika* (1942) **32**, 101–27, 203–25, and **33**, 1–24.

Bronowski's observation is in *A Sense of the Future* (1977), M.I.T. Press.

For Venn's definition see Further Reading: *The Logic of Chance.*

The research questions analogy is from Kurman in *Et Cetera* (1977) **34**, 265–76.

CHAPTER 3

For the distinction between pragmatic and explanatory emphasis see Schwartz and others in Further Reading: *Clinical Trials.*

For Venn's analogy see Further Reading: *The Logic of Chance.*

The estimation of proportions histogram and calculations are based on Mainland's sampling experiment, see *Elementary Medical Statistics* (1952), Saunders.

For Murphy's comment see Further Reading: *The Logic of Medicine.*

For Sackett's list of biases see *Journal of Chronic Diseases* (1979) **32,** 51–63.

Data in the proportions of babies table are from Kinsey and Zacharias in *J.A.M.A.* (1949) **139,** 572–8.

The tuberculosis treatment trial is described in Hill's *Statistical Methods in Clinical and Preventive Medicine* (1962), Oxford Univ. Press.

The national RLF trial details are given by Kinsey in *Arch. Ophthalmol.* (1956) **56,** 481–543.

The cancer risk data are from Bibbo and others in *N. Eng. J. Med.* (1978) **298,** 763–7.

Tukey's comments appear in his article in *Science* (1977) **198,** 679–84.

CHAPTER 4

The looking backward comment of Schneiderman is in *Am. J. Roent.* (1966) **96,** 230–55.

The scarlet fever and tuberculosis trends are redrawn (with permission) from McKeown's *The Modern Rise of Population* (1976), Edward Arnold.

The tuberculosis treatment trial is described in Hill's *Statistical Methods in Clinical and Preventive Medicine* (1962), Oxford Univ. Press.

Shifts in distribution of births is described by Morris in *Am. J. Pub. Health* (1975) **65,** 359–62.

Odell's discovery is reported in *Pediatrics* (1959) **55,** 268–79.

Wesley's drawing of lots is quoted by David in *Games, Gods and Gambling* (1962), Charles Griffen and Co.

The print of Leombruno's painting is from Pinacoteca di Brera, Milan.

Fisher's explanation appears in his original textbook *Statistical Methods for Research Workers* (1925), Oliver and Boyd.

The advantages of random allotment are discussed by Byar and co-workers in *N. Eng. J. Med.* (1976) **295,** 74–80.

Prognostic stratification is discussed by Peto and others, see Further Readings: *Design and . . .*

Chalmer's proposal appears in *Med. Clin. N. Am.* (1975) **59**, 1035–8.

The experience of surgical treatment to prevent esophageal hemorrhage is summarized by Grace and others in *Gastroenterology* (1966) **50**, 684–91 and revised (copyright 1977 AAAS) by Gilbert and others in *Science* (1977) **198**, 684–9.

Play the winner plan is described by Zelen in *J. Am. Stat. Assoc.* (1969) **64**, 131–45.

For the 'two armed bandit' approach see Weinstein in *N. Eng. J. Med.* (1974) **291**, 1278–85.

CHAPTER 5

The national RLF trial details are given by Kinsey in *Arch. Ophthalmol.* (1956) **56**, 481–543.

The wide range of outcomes bar graph is redrawn (with permission) from Fielding and others in *Lancet* (1978) **ii**, 778–9.

For Peto's comments concerning planning trials see Further Reading: *Design and . . .*

For details of the ACTH experience see Further Reading: *Retrolental . . .*

Oxygen dosage in the national RLF trial is given by Kinsey in *Arch. Ophthalmol.* (1956) **56**, 481–543.

The cerebral palsy and RLF frequencies are from McDonald in *Arch. Dis. Childhood* (1963) **38**, 579–88.

The influences of experimenters are discussed by Rosenthal in his book *Experimenter's Effects in Behavioral Research* (1976), Irvington, and in *Et Cetera* (1977) **34**, 253–64.

Wolf's account of a placebo effect in asthma is in *Proc. Ass. Res. Nerv. Mental Dis.* (1959) **37**, 147–61.

Conditional trial design is discussed by Feinstein, see Further Reading: *Clinical Biostatistics.*

The list of biases is from Sackett in *J. Chron. Dis.* (1979) **32**, 51–63.

CHAPTER 6

Dobson's observation is from Asher's lectures in *Trans. Med. Soc. Lond.* (1959) **75**, 66–72.

Doctor Bell's observations and preliminary notes on Sherlock Holmes are from Michael and Mollie Hardwick's *The Man who was Sherlock Holmes* (1964), John Murray.

The announcement of topics and the Hidden Man figures are from Asher's lectures printed in *Trans. Med. Soc. Lond.* (1959) **75**, 66–72.

Recording errors in behavioral research are noted by Rosenthal in his book *Experimenter's Effects in Behavioral Research* (1976), Irvington.

Properties of sets of measurements are discussed by Youden in *Sci. Monthly* (1953) **76**, 143–7.

CHAPTER 7

The death and survival with handicap bar graph is redrawn (with permission) from Kitchen and others in *Dev. Med. Child Neurol.* (1979) **21**, 582–9.

Assessments in surgical treatments are reported by Gilbert and co-workers in *Science* (1977) **198**, 684–9.

The cusum line graph is redrawn (with permission) from Wohl in *N. Eng. J. Med.* (1977) **296**, 1044–45.

The Rumplestiltskin effect is from Asher in *Trans. Med. Soc. Lond.* (1959) **75**, 66–72.

The chance difference in mortality figure is redrawn (with permission) from Peto and others, see Further Reading: *Design and* ...

CHAPTER 8

For Murphy's story about confoundment see Further Reading: *The Logic of Medicine*.

Calculation of standardized event rates is explained by Hill in *Principles of Medical Statistics* (1966), Oxford Univ. Press. For Feinstein's examples of unequal prognoses and unequal compliance see Further Reading: *Clinical Biostatistics*.

Mainland's guidelines are in *J. Chron. Dis.* (1960) **11**, 480–96.

The exclusions ... figure is redrawn (with permission) from Peto and others, see Further Reading: *Design and* ...

The clinical trial committee suggestions are Klimt's, see *Cont. Clin. Trials* (1981) **1**, 283–93.

CHAPTER 9

Positive-pressure treatment is described by Gregory and others in *N. Eng. J. Med.* (1971) **284**, 1333–40.

The idealized model of diagnosis is redrawn (with permission) from Card and Good, see Further Reading: *A Logical Analysis* ...

The role of hypothesis testing in clinical trials is discussed in reports of a biometrics seminar, see *J. Chron. Dis.* (1966) **19,** 857–82.

The number of patients to enroll figures are redrawn (with permission) from Clark and Downie in *Lancet* (1966) **ii,** 1357–8.

Freiman and collaborators' review of negative trials is in *N. Eng. J. Med.* (1978) **299,** 690–4.

Data in the high versus low oxygen table are from Lanman and others in the *J.A.M.A.* (1954) **155,** 223–6.

The 'peeking' problem bar graph (redrawn with permission) and the adjusted significance levels are from McPherson in *N. Eng. J. Med.* (1974) **290,** 501–2.

CHAPTER 10

The roles of Pearson and Fisher are discussed by Mainland in *Clin. Pharm. Therap.* (1963) **4,** 580–6.

The single hospital experiment results are from Lanman and others in *J.A.M.A.* (1954) **155,** 223–6.

The number of trials table is from Peto and others, see Further Reading: *Design and* . . .

The publication decisions story is from Hudson's *A Case of Need* (1968), New American Library.

Sterling's arguments are in *J.A. Stat. Assoc.* (1959) **54,** 30–6.

The probabilities in the multiplicity of classes bar graph (copyright 1977 AAAS) are from Tukey in *Science* (1977) **198,** 679–84.

Statistical proof is discussed by Darlington, see Further Reading: *Radicals and* . . .

The Bayesian example is based on Mainland's discussion in *Clin. Pharm. Therap.* (1967) **8,** 738–48.

For Darlington's suggestion about the interpretation of 'significance' see Further Reading: *Radicals and* . . .

Smithell's comment is in *Arch. Dis. Childhood* (1978) **53,** 604–7.

CHAPTER 11

Cardano's portrait is from the Bettman Archive.

Shapiro's evaluation of clinical predictions is in *N. Eng. J. Med.* (1977) **296,** 1509–14.

Formulation of a decision problem is from Raiffa's *Decision Analysis: Introductory Lectures on Choices Under Uncertainty* (1968), Addison-Wesley.

Decision theory terms and a medical decision model (redrawn with permission) are from Card and Good, see Further Reading: *A Logical Analysis* ...

The benefits and costs figure is redrawn (with permission) from Pauker and Kassirer in *N. Eng. J. Med.* (1975) **293**, 229–34.

Subjective judgment is discussed by Raiffa in *Decision Analysis* ... (1968), Addison-Wesley.

Fisher's comment is quoted by Mainland in *Clin. Pharm. Therap.* (1960) **1**, 411–22.

Mahler's reasoning appears in *WHO Chron.* (1977) **31**, 8–12.

'Evangelists' and 'snails' are compared by Sackett in *Lancet* (1975) **ii**, 357–61.

Mumford's comment is in *Values for Survival* (1946), Brace and Co.

CHAPTER 12

A modified version of this chapter appeared in *Persp. Biol. Med.* (1983) **26**, 343–53.

Haggard's description of the treatment of King Charles is from *Devils, Drugs and Doctors* (1929), Harper.

The proliferation of codes is discussed by Katz in a report to H.E.W. Assistant Secretary for Health, M.K. Duval (unpublished, dated 1973).

The cancer cells incident is described in Katz's *Experimentation with Human Beings* (1972), Russell Sage Foundation.

Comroe and Dripps review is in *Science* (1976) **192**, 105–11.

Rabi's comment is in *The Nature of Scientific Discovery* (1975, Owen Gingerich, editor), Smithsonian Institution Press.

Dworkin's definitions are in his book, see Further Reading: *Taking Rights* ...

Sigerist's comments about the people's health are from *Medicine and Human Welfare* (1941), Yale Univ. Press.

The outcomes in trials data (copyright 1977 AAAS) are from Gilbert and co-workers in *Science* (1977) **198**, 684–9.

The findings of the National Institutes of Health task force are reported by Cardon and others in *N. Eng. J. Med.* (1976) **295**, 650–4.

Cassileth and co-workers' findings are in *J.A.M.A.* (1982) **248**, 968–70.

The National Commission ... recommendations are discussed by Levine, see Further Reading: *Ethics and Regulation*.

Jonas' reflections are in *Daedalus* (1969) **219**, 235–41.

Eisenberg's comments are in *Science* (1977) **198**, 1105–8.

Preliminary data in Simes and Tattersall's survey are cited in *B.M.J.* (1983) **286**, 1972–3.

Chalmers' findings are in *Mt Sinai J. Med.* (1974) **41**, 753–8.

For Freidson's comments see Further Reading: *The Profession* ...

For Popper's parable see Further Reading: *Conjectures* ...

APPENDIX A

For details of the RLF story see Further Reading: *Retrolental* ...

APPENDIX B

The check list for randomized trials is from Chalmers and others in *Cont. Clin. Trials* (1981) **2**, 31–49.

Index

Abbreviations after page numbers: ac = acknowledgments and citations; ap = appendix; b = boxed comments; f = figure; fr = further reading; t = table.

in polio trials, 165
see also sampling
reproducibility of observations, 92–5
research
  in agriculture, 10–11b, 26
  basic biomedical, 158–9
  goal directed, 158, 159
  guidelines (FDA), 151b
  'purposeless', 158
  questions in, 14–29
  see also experiments; trials
respirations, oxygen and, 55, 60
retrolental fibroplasia, *see* RLF
review committees, 158
review, prior, 157–8
rights
  abstract, 160
  concrete, 160–61
  of dissent, 168
  of health, 159–60
risks, *see* trials, risk in; trials, risk
  limitation in
risk and benefit evaluation, 162–3
  'significance' level and, 130
  see also decision analysis, benefits
  and costs format
RLF
  ACTH and, 59–60, 175ap
  in animals, 61, 176ap
  birth weight and, 35t, 36f, 51f
  blood transfusions and, 18
  Boston survey of, 16–17, 18, 19,
    174ap
  'causes' of, speculated, 174ap
  in cities, 35t, 173ap
  congenital, 24b
  follow-up of, 177–8ap
  in hospitals, 16–19, 35t
  important difference in frequency,
    121
  incubators and, 175ap
  iron administration and, 16–17,
    174ap
  in Melbourne, 18–19, 22, 135b,
    175ap
  national trial, *see* multicenter trials,
    of oxygen
  oxygen and, *see* oxygen, and RLF
  resurgence of, 179ap
  retrospective surveys of, 35t, 173ap
  stages of, 79
  story of, *viii*, 173–9ap

and strawberry marks, 102
and survival, 122t
twins and, 77
in the US (general), 174ap, 176ap
vitamins and, 16–17, 174–5ap
without oxygen treatment, 24b, 178ap
Rosenthal, R., 64f, 65b, 188ac
roulette, 99
Rumpelstiltskin effect, 94b
Rutstein, David, 165b

Sackett D.L.
  on biases, 34b, 68b, 187ac
  influence of, 12
  on pace of innovation, 149, 191ac
  on reading journals, 183fr
sample size graphs, 117f, 118f
sampling
  assumptions in, 31
  in clinical studies, 33–8
  haphazard, 33
  random, 30–31, 32–3b
scales of measurement, 77–80
scarlet fever, 43
scandals, 157
Schneiderman, M.A., 42, 187ac
Schwartz, D., 30, 182fr
science
  advances in, 158–9
  criticism in, *ix*, 8
  freedom of inquiry in, 158–9
  method, basic tenet of, 18
  objectivity of, 171
  rules of evidence, hardship and, 8
  social aspect of, 171–2
  values of, 159
  see also Popper, Karl R.
scores, for signs and symptoms, 79–80
scurvy, 7b
Selvin, H.C., 20, 186ac
semiology, medical, 71
sensitivity
  of a test, 95b
  of trials, 50
sequential analysis, 125
  see also multiple look issue
sham procedure, 66
Shapiro, A.R., 141–2, 190ac
Sigerist, Henry E., 161b, 191ac
'significance'
  belief and, 137
  confusion about, 127–8